TAKING MY PLACE IN MEDICINE

This book is dedicated to my husband Jerry
and my sons Jerry and Joel.
You are my world.

TAKING MY PLACE IN MEDICINE

CARMEN WEBB
EDITOR

A Guide for Minority Medical Students

Sage Publications, Inc.
International Educational and Professional Publisher
Thousand Oaks ▪ London ▪ New Delhi

For information:

Sage Publications, Inc.
2455 Teller Road
Thousand Oaks, California 91320
E-mail: order@sagepub.com

Sage Publications Ltd.
6 Bonhill Street
London EC2A 4PU
United Kingdom

Sage Publications India Pvt. Ltd.
M-32 Market
Greater Kailash I
New Delhi 110 048 India

Printed in the United States of America

Library of Congress Cataloging-in-Publication Data

Main entry under title:

  Taking my place in medicine: A guide for minority medical students / edited by Carmen Webb.
    p.   cm.—(Surviving medical school; v. 8)
  Includes bibliographical references and index.
  ISBN 0-7619-1809-4 (pbk.: alk. paper)
  1. Minorities in medicine—United States.   2. Medical students—United States.   3. Medical education—United States.   I. Webb, Carmen.
  II. Series.
  R693 .M57   2000
  610'71'173 dc21   00-008370

This book is printed on acid-free paper.

00   01   02   03   04   05   06   7   6   5   4   3   2   1

Acquiring Editors:	Rolf Janke/Jim Nageotte
Editorial Assistant:	Heidi Van Middlesworth
Production Editor:	Astrid Virding
Editorial Assistant:	Victoria Cheng
Copyeditor:	Linda Gray
Typesetter:	Lynn Miyata
Indexer:	Kathy Paparchontis

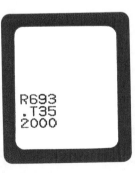

Contents

Foreword   ix

Preface   xiii

Introduction   xvii
    A Word About Language   xviii
    A More Personal Word   xix
    Acknowledgments   xix

How to Use This Book   xxi

Section I. Navigating a New World   **1**

1. Medical Culture   **3**
    Ana E. Núñez, MD
    Exactly Who Am I?   3
    What Is This Place?   5
    Taking My Place Within the Culture of Medicine   14
    Conclusion   16
    Sample Conflicts   17

2. Mastering the First Two Years   **22**
    Carmen Webb, MD, and Morris Hawkins, Jr., PhD
    Preparing Yourself   22

In the Classroom   23
In the Labs   24
What If My Way Doesn't Work Anymore?   26
Balance: How Is It Possible?   27
How Do I Not Feel Guilty for Relaxation Time?   32
Managing Competition   33
Maintaining Motivation   35
The USMLE: Meeting "Standardized" Challenges   39
Conclusion   44

3. Life on the Wards: When All the Rules Change   **45**
   Margarita Hauser Gardiner, MD

PART I: THE NEW RULES

Clinical Clerkships   46
Who's Who   47
The Daily Routine   49
Student Responsibilities   50

PART II: WHEN THINGS GO WRONG

Stumbling Blocks   53
Effective Defensive Strategies   58

4. Now What Will I Do? Preparing for Residency   **63**
   Carmen Webb, MD

Choosing a Specialty   63
Mastering the Process   69
Conclusion   76

Section II. Focus on Me   **79**

5. Do I Really Belong Here?   **81**
   Carmen Webb, MD

Myths About Minorities   81
Impact of the Myths   86
Realistic Self-Appraisal   88
Conclusion   94

6. Taking Care of Myself   **97**
Carmen Webb, MD

Taking Stock   97

Understanding My Needs   98

Making a Plan   103

Designing Personalized Methods of Coping With Stress   107

Conclusion   116

7. Building a Community   **119**
Carmen Webb, MD, and George C. Gardiner, MD

The Problem: Isolation   119

Choosing My Crowd   121

The Role of the Office of Minority Affairs in My Community   125

Finding Mentors in My Community   127

The Family in Your Community: A Balancing Act   130

Conclusion   135

Section III. Focus on My Culture   **137**

8. Focus on African American Medical Students   **139**
Carmen Webb, MD, Stephanie Smith,
Morris Hawkins, Jr., PhD, and Ann Hill, MEd

History of African Americans in Medicine   139

Current Status   142

Special Challenges   144

Secrets of Success: Advice From Fifty Black Physicians   147

What African Americans Offer the World of Medicine   151

Conclusion   152

9. Focus on Native American Medical Students   **156**
Lori Arviso Alvord, MD

History of Native Americans in Medicine   156

Current Status   158

Special Challenges   158

Secrets of Success for Native American Students   166

What Native Americans Offer the World of Medicine   167

10. Focus on Mexican American Medical Students   **172**
    Miguel A. Bedolla, MD, PhD, MPH

    History of Mexican Americans in Medicine   173
    Current Status   174
    Special Challenges   175
    Secrets of Success   181
    What Mexican Americans Offer the World of Medicine   184

11. Focus on Puerto Rican Medical Students   **186**
    Maria Soto-Greene, MD, and Juan C. Martínez, MD

    History of Puerto Ricans in Medicine   187
    Current Status   187
    Special Challenges   188
    Secrets of Success and Survival   194
    What Puerto Ricans Offer the World of Medicine   195
    Conclusion   195

12. Managing Racism   **198**
    Kevin Bakeer Al-Mateen, MD, and Cheryl S. Al-Mateen, MD

    Historical Perspectives   199
    Psychology of Racism   200
    Racism on Campus   201
    Impact on the Victim   202
    Intervention Strategies   203
    Making Your Case   206
    Summary   209
    Discussion Vignettes   209

Afterword   213

Author Index   215

Subject Index   219

About the Editor   224

About the Contributors   226

Foreword

Adapting to life as a medical trainee challenges any student. Minority students—African Americans, Mexican Americans, Native Americans, Mainland Puerto Ricans, and Hawaiians—whose backgrounds often differ from those who govern medical centers, need also to adapt to the values, beliefs, and customs of the dominant group. Mentors with similar backgrounds, who can serve as role models, are usually sorely lacking.

This book is designed to help minority students thrive personally and academically in medical school, to make a realistic assessment of their strengths and weaknesses, to successfully confront societal myths and stereotypes, and to develop healthy strategies to meet academic, personal, and relationship needs. Dr. Carmen Webb, having assisted countless medical students with these very issues, has assembled an outstanding cadre of insightful professionals to address these important needs. Each contributor is highly qualified and devoted to promoting medical student well-being.

Carmen Webb, MD, Adjunct Assistant Professor of Psychiatry at MCP Hahnemann School of Medicine (MCPHU) in Philadelphia, is currently practicing in Dallas, Texas. She established the first Medical Student Mental Health Service at MCPHU and teaches courses and workshops to help minority students develop the skills needed to survive medical school. As principal investigator of a multi-institutional study, she evaluated the psychosocial characteristics and skills that predict academic performance in medical school across race and gender.

Cheryl S. Al-Mateen, MD, a Forensic Child and Adolescent Psychiatrist at the Virginia Commonwealth University's Medical College of Virginia (VCU), is also a faculty associate at the Institute for Law, Psychiatry and Public Policy at the University of Virginia. Her publications and presentations focus on cultural competence, sexuality, identity development, and mental health of African American women. She has also conducted research on the effects of community violence on children and adolescents. She has long been adviser, supervisor, and mentor to premedical and medical students.

Kevin Bakeer Al-Mateen, MD, MSHA, a neonatologist at the Virginia Commonwealth University's Medical College of Virginia (VCU), also holds a master's degree in health administration. A member of the Committee on the Status of Women and Minorities in Medicine at VCU, he is a faculty adviser and mentor to residents and medical students.

Lori Arviso Alvord, MD, a board-certified surgeon and Associate Dean of Student Affairs and Minority Affairs at Dartmouth Medical School, is one of the most accomplished Native Americans in medicine today. She oversees admissions, financial aid, student affairs, and minority affairs. An enrolled member of the Navajo Tribe, she spent six years working with the Public Health Service among Navajo and Zuni tribes in Gallup, New Mexico.

Miguel A. Bedolla, MD, PhD, MPH, Associate Professor of Family Practice at the University of Texas Health Science Center in San Antonio and Charles Miller Professor of Medical Ethics at St. Mary's University, is the Director of the South Texas/Border Region Partnership for Health Professions Education. This program, with others, is dedicated to offering minority applicants equal opportunities to attend Texas medical schools.

George C. Gardiner, MD, board certified in internal medicine and psychiatry, has recruited, trained, and counseled medical students for 30 years. As Associate Provost of Minority Affairs at MCP Hahnemann School of Medicine at Allegheny University of the Health Sciences, his department recruited the largest number of minority students at any majority medical school. Most recently, he served as Clinical Director for the Dr. Warren E. Smith Health Centers in Philadelphia.

Margarita Hauser Gardiner, MD, board certified in Internal Medicine and Rheumatology, is on faculty at MCP Hahnemann School of Medicine where she advised, mentored, and served as clinical preceptor for second-, third-, and fourth-year medical students. Currently working with a pharmaceutical company as a drug safety monitor, she continues to supervise and mentor premedical and medical students.

Morris Hawkins, Jr., PhD, Associate Professor of Cell Biology and Molecular Genetics and Special Assistant to the Dean of Howard University College of Medicine, is a research adviser, mentor, and support to undergraduate, medical, and doctoral students. He coordinates the Liaison Committee on Medical Education Self-Study Accreditation site visits for the College of Medicine, was Vice Chairman of the Middle State University-wide Self Study for Accreditation, and Chaired the NCAA Self-Study for Athletics Certification.

Ann Hill, MEd, served as past Director of Minority Affairs at MCPHU, and past Assistant Professor and Assistant Director of Admissions at Cheyney University of Pennsylvania. In her role, she was responsible for recruitment and admissions of minority medical students and for assisting them in developing strategies for academic success. As director of the freshman studies program, she assisted students in developing strategies for academic success.

Juan C. Martinez, EdD, Senior Educational Planner at UMDNJ-New Jersey Medical School, has been involved in academic advising and curricular development for over 20 years. He coordinates support services, conducts cognitive development sessions for first- and second-year students, and performs follow-up evaluations on student examination performance, particularly for underrepresented minority students.

Ana Núñez, MD, Assistant Professor of Medicine, Assistant Dean for Generalism, and Director of the Women's Health Education Program at MCPHU, is a member of the National Advisory to the Robert Wood Johnson, Minority Medical Education Program. She edits a comprehensive women's health case study series, is principal investigator of a U.S. Department of Education grant, and has nationally recognized expertise in cross-cultural communication and cultural diversity issues.

Maria Soto-Greene, MD, Acting Associate Dean for Special Programs at the New Jersey Medical School, has more than a dozen years of experience with minority issues, especially among Puerto Ricans. She is board certified in Internal Medicine, Critical Care, and Emergency Medicine. She is principal investigator of a federally funded program to increase the number of Hispanic/

Latino physicians who can favorably affect the health and well-being of their communities.

Stephanie Smith, currently a third-year medical student at Virginia Commonwealth University's Medical College of Virginia, completed her first two years of medical education at MCPHU where she was honored as a Humanities Scholar and was involved in the Student National Medical Association (SNMA), the Holistic Medicine Society, Pen Friends, and several outreach programs.

—Robert Holman Coombs
Professor of Biobehavioral Science, UCLA School of Medicine
Series Editor

—Carla Cronkhite Vera
Department of Psychiatry, UCLA School of Medicine

Preface

In the early 1950s, I was elated when granted an interview at the University of Virginia College of Medicine. Although I was an A student and a native of Virginia, I was turned down for admission. The rejection was not surprising because in that era, African American admissions to Virginia medical schools were virtually nonexistent. I subsequently sought and was afforded admission to Meharry Medical College in Nashville, Tennessee. As a graduate, I still cherish the fact that Meharry, along with Howard University Medical School, Washington, D.C., was there for me and for thousands of other African Americans, many of whom were denied admission to publicly funded Anglo medical schools.

Twenty years later, as a busy physician practicing in San Antonio, I was greatly concerned that admissions rates for minorities remained dismally low. Therefore, I was delighted to accept an invitation by the University of Texas Health Science Center, San Antonio, to serve as an advocate for minorities on its medical school admissions committee. For some six years, I participated with other members of diverse ethnicity who shared the same urgency to improve minority admission rates. We identified many excellent minority candidates who would otherwise have "fallen through the cracks" and not been granted admission.

It became obvious that the medical schools who are competitive in enrolling and *graduating* minority medical students must effectively meet two challenges: (a) to provide at the personal level a "user-friendly" environment for entering minority medical students and (b) to forearm them with sufficient insight, guidelines, and strategies to ensure their success in medical school, despite ethnic adversities. With the publication of this book titled *Taking My Place in Medicine: A Guide for Minority Medical Students,* both medical schools and their minority medical students are fortunate to have a powerful resource to help meet these challenges.

The book is a stellar work conceived by one author and made powerful by its diversity of coauthors. It is destined to have broad readership throughout the medical community and beyond. Written primarily to benefit minority medical students, this work will serve as an invaluable navigational guide as they embark on a formidable voyage in pursuit of excellence. It deals candidly with a broad range of expected concerns of minority medical students entering the medical arena.

This book begins by providing minority medical students with a comprehensive definition of the established medical culture, including the language, structure, traditions, and challenges this culture presents to minorities. Through the eyes of the authors, minority medical students will see medical school life in its stark reality. Without personal bias, the authors leave no stone unturned as they expose the "minefields," "roadblocks," and other hazards peculiarly encountered by non-Anglo medical students. Thought-provoking illustrations and vignettes provide dynamic realism as well as clarity to this work.

Early on, minority medical students are challenged to make a realistic self-appraisal of their inner strengths and to assess the medical and nonmedical support systems available. They are brought face to face with cultural myths with which they must deal, lest these myths become self-defeating.

As students progress from the classroom and labs of the basic science years to the bedside of the clinical years to local and national examinations and, subsequently, to matching for residencies, challenges vary but not the anxieties they bring. The varieties of difficulties are carefully presented as potential adversities that, with foreknowledge, can be largely attenuated. Available strategies for staying the course, surviving, and overcoming are carefully charted. The positive, can-do approach to managing challenges, small and great alike, is refreshing and, for the student, encouraging. Indeed, minority medical students are admonished to strive for excellence, to persevere, and to maintain an attitude of professionalism, despite adversity.

The chapters dealing with specific ethnic concerns are especially valuable as they provide an up-close look at each of the following cultural groups: African American, Mexican American, Native American, and Puerto Rican. Authors ethnically and culturally related to these groups provide the great wealth of information covered. Each author has taken pains to present a candid historical review of conflicts previously encountered in the medical school setting along with strategies for management. Thus, the minority student from any of these cultural groups is treated to a "customized" view of problems peculiar to his or her specific group. Challenges common to all groups are presented, but management strategies and "secrets" to success vary from group to group. It is made clear that not all conflicts can be managed simply as "Black versus White" issues.

"Managing Racism" is masterfully addressed in the final chapter. Its scholarly definition of the issues in historical context shares much-needed wisdom regarding the perpetrators as well as the victims of racism in the medical arena. The appropriate response of the victim, depending on type of injury and local support structure available, is skillfully presented. These well-referenced pages are notably free of bias and have provided for minority medical students a splendid "road map" from victim to victory.

Dr. Webb and the contributing authors are to be congratulated for this valuable work so rich in insight and dedication to detail. It adds considerable depth to our understanding of an area of medical education that has previously been afforded far too little attention. The book stands out as a remarkable single-source reference for minority medical students, medical school deans, faculty, admissions committees, and medical career counselors. All are privileged to have this volume and are profoundly indebted to the authors.

—Charles S. Thurston, MD
Department of Medicine/Dermatology,
University of Texas Health Science Center

Introduction

Any student working to succeed in medicine navigates a whole new culture. You will be no exception. In addition to the academics, you must master the language, values, beliefs, and customs particular to medical school—because much of the medical world is based on historically White Western male values. Adapting to this culture can be challenging for any student, and particularly challenging for you who, as a minority student, often do not share these mores. Furthermore, for groups historically underrepresented in the field, knowledge about how to achieve in medicine may not be readily available. In other words, you may not have anyone to coach you in the "rules of the system." However, your understanding of these expectations is critical to your success.

In addition to understanding the system, to thrive personally and academically in medical school, you must make a realistic assessment of your abilities. This includes screening out the myths and stereotypes imposed by society. You also must develop healthy strategies to meet your academic, personal, and relational needs. Although minority students share many similar experiences within the medical school system, they are in no way a homogeneous group. African Americans, Native Americans, Puerto Rican Americans, and Mexican Americans differ significantly. In addition, there are critical cultural differences within each ethnic group. Understanding the possible impact of cultural heritage on your medical school experience, including the impact of racism, is extremely important.

Our purpose in this book is to help you to (a) understand the medical school culture and expectations, (b) identify strategies that will meet your personal and academic needs, and (c) address the specific challenges arising from the interface of your ethnic heritage and medical school culture.

A Word About Language

The term *minority* is often used to include many groups (gender, age, sexual preference) who are not part of the majority in the United States. In this book, we use the word interchangeably with *ethnic minority,* and our focus will be ethnic groups historically underrepresented in U.S. medical schools. According to the Association of American Medical Colleges (AAMC), these groups include Blacks (African Americans), Native Americans, Mexican Americans, and Puerto Ricans. Certainly, there are many other groups who face challenges in medical school because of their nonmajority status (e.g., Asian Americans). However, because we are not able to address all ethnic groups effectively in one short book, we have chosen to focus on those who are historically underrepresented. (We suspect that much of the information will be useful to other students who are not part of the majority.)

We will use the terms *Black* and *African American* interchangeably. Using the Health Resources and Services Administration (HRSA) definition, these terms will refer to all Black Americans "having origin in any of the Black racial groups of Africa." This includes all Black Americans of African descent, including Caribbean Americans. The term *Native American* will refer to an individual who is a member of a tribe of people (living in the United States) indigenous to the Americas. We use the terms *Puerto Rican* and *Puerto Rican Mainland* interchangeably. Puerto Rican Mainland refers to persons from Puerto Rico who reside in the United States. *Mexican American* refers to persons having origin in Mexico who are now American citizens. *Hispanic* or *Latino* will connote all Puerto Rican or Mexican American persons.

This book addresses the interface between medical culture, personal values and beliefs, and ethnic culture. We hope that it will be an invaluable tool for all minority students striving to take their places in medicine.

A More Personal Word

I love practicing medicine. Psychiatry is the perfect match for me. But when I look around, I am lonely for more minority colleagues. Over the past 13 years, I've worked with students who are striving to get through medical school. I am constantly struck by how much not knowing the system contributes to their distress. You just don't want to waste time struggling with medical culture when you could be learning medicine (or otherwise living the rest of your life).

My personal hope for this book is that it will give you and other minority students a road map to navigate the system. Although we've told many of the stories of minority students here, we have undoubtedly left out some. If yours is yet unrecorded, take pen in hand. We need to hear your wisdom.

I want the minority student who reads this to be empowered to move through the medical world with confidence—not just surviving but thriving. As the title indicates, you have a place in medicine: It's your responsibility to step up and take it.

Acknowledgments

My first and greatest thanks goes to God, who has given me this work, knowing that I would love it, knowing the timing was perfect. He provided me with the personal dedication and the editorial, emotional, and mentoring support that I needed and has guided me every step of the way.

I give special thanks to Diane Cohen, a wonderful friend, who has read every word, almost as many times as I have. She has been unyielding in her standards for excellence as we tightened the language of this manuscript. Equally important, she has given her moral support and encouragement.

Thanks to all the contributing authors, who are marvelous writers and who provided much of the content that made this book possible. I count them among my most respected colleagues. Special thanks to Kevin Bakeer Al-Mateen, MD, who reviewed the entire manuscript.

This book reflects the support of many other family members and friends. For helpful editorial comments, I thank Drew Alexander; Cynthia Baker;

Rickie Baker; Davida Bolger; Patti Cooper; Lonnie Fuller, Sr., MD; Benjamin Gallman, Esq.; Lisa George, Esq.; Linda Hiner, MD; Kempton Ingersol; Romaine Johnson, MD; Linda Mitchell; Reggie Moore, MD; Renee Moore; Kim Mueser, PhD; Liz Noll; Valerie Patton; William Sedlacek, PhD; Jerry Webb, MD; and Vincent Zarro, MD; and for motivation, Rev. Steven Lawrence. I am very appreciative of the insightful comments shared by College of Medicine students at Howard University. I would also like to thank the students with whom I have worked over the years for sharing their lives and innumerable experiences with me.

I thank Bob Coombs, PhD, whose vision and care for medical students made this happen.

My loving gratitude goes to Jerry Webb, MD, my husband, who was my greatest support through medical school. He has patiently supported me in this work also, giving me excellent ideas and sacrificing often so that I might complete this manuscript. I am deeply indebted to Cynthia and Rickie Baker; Patti and Paul Cooper; Renee Moore; Reggie Moore, MD; Tracy, Kelly, Jennifer, Jessica, Paige, and Michelle; Gertrude and Lee Snell; Tonya Ingersol; and Lucille Lawrence, all of whom helped simplify my life so I could get the work done.

I especially thank my in-laws, Joseph and Betty Culberson, Tricia Webb (whose own book is coming out soon), Tangela Pollack, Brian Shields, Walter and Doris Reed, Egypt Allen, Terry Webb, Theresa Enoch, and all the other Webbs by birth or marriage who worked tirelessly to help us relocate while I worked on this book.

Finally, I thank my parents. Marie Thurston, now pursuing her own doctorate at the age of 68, is my model of a strong and courageous woman. I savor her unwavering support and encouragement. Charles Thurston, MD, the first physician I ever met, has provided me with an example of a smart and compassionate doctor. Because of him, I've never had to question whether African Americans have a place in medicine.

How to Use This Book

As you open this book, you will encounter the challenges and joys that you as a minority student face in medical training. Remember, however, that this is not meant to be an exhaustive manual. It is one in a series of books that provide in-depth looks at life as a medical student. You may choose to read this volume cover to cover or to use it as a reference for the issues that arise during your journey. If you plan to take it a few chapters at a time, the following may help you find the sections most pertinent to your needs.

Premedical and First-Year Students. To ready yourself for the medical world, begin with the chapters "Medical Culture" (Chapter 1), "Mastering the First Two Years" (Chapter 2), and "Taking Care of Myself" (Chapter 6). These will give you a leg up on managing first encounters with ease.

Second-Year Students. You will want to focus on "Life on the Wards" (Chapter 3) and to reread the USMLE section of Chapter 2. These chapters will help you to position yourself for the boards and for the clinical years ahead.

Third- and Fourth-Year Students. You will find it useful to read "Now What Will I Do" (Chapter 4) and the "Realistic Self-Appraisal" section of Chapter 5. Reread "Life on the Wards" (Chapter 3) and the "The Rules" section of Chapter 1. These chapters will remind you of the new expectations in the clinical years and prepare you for the challenge of finding the best residency for your own career.

All Years. When you are having doubts about your abilities, your potential or your future, read "Do I Really Belong Here?" (Chapter 5). When racist attitudes or cultural hurdles arise, read "Managing Racism" (Chapter 12) and the appropriate "Focus on My Culture" sections. As you struggle with maintaining a fulfilling life while dealing with medical school, pick up "Taking Care of Myself" (Chapter 6) and "Building a Community" (Chapter 7); also, reread the section on "Balance" in Chapter 2.

Faculty. To understand the challenges of your minority students in the classroom and on the floors, peruse the chapters "Mastering the First Two Years" (Chapter 2) and "Life on the Wards" (Chapter 3). Those of you teaching classes in cross-cultural issues or medical culture will find a wonderful resource in "Medical Culture" (Chapter 1) or the chapters in "Focus on My Culture" (Section III).

Premed Advisers, Faculty Advisers, Summer Program Directors, Student Affairs Personnel, Student Support, and Mental Health Personnel. As you work to understand and guide students of all ethnicities through their daily hurdles, use this book for your own reference or recommend pertinent sections to your students. The chapters "Medical Culture" (Chapter 1) and "Building a Community" (Chapter 7) may be especially helpful during orientation periods. When preparing students for the changing expectations of the curriculum, you may recommend "Mastering the First Two Years" (Chapter 2), "Life on the Wards" (Chapter 3), and "Now What Will I Do?" (Chapter 4.) When helping a student to adjust to the rigorous demands of medical school, you may find especially helpful the chapters on "Taking Care of Myself" (Chapter 6) and "Do I Really Belong Here?" (Chapter 5). The "Focus on My Culture" section (Section III) may help students to place their challenges in context and to prepare for a diverse medical world.

Section I
Navigating a New World

When at last you open that acceptance letter to medical school, what can you expect? What will the medical school experience *be* like? And how will it be for you as a minority student? The next four chapters will help you understand the culture of this brand new world. We will point out landmarks (and land mines) and suggest tools to help you to navigate the basic science and clinical years. We also offer tips for managing the process of your securing the best residency for you.

1 Medical Culture

ANA E. NÚÑEZ, MD

Training in medicine is an induction into a new world. The challenges of becoming a physician enable you to grow, to learn more about yourself and others, and to test your strength of character. The world of medicine has its own traditions, values, beliefs, dress, and language. The sooner you understand what they are, what they mean, and what is valued, the easier you can assess how to fit into this world.

Exactly Who Am I?

Most people entering medical school are at a developmental age in which they are crafting their initial adult identity. How aware are you of the influences of your ethnicity, your gender, your family? If you haven't thought about it much yet, consider it now. Identity development is fluid. Reflection and awareness help us craft an intentional being rather than being buffeted about by situations or taking all experiences in without using healthy filters. What do you value? What traditions are important to you? What values do you reject? Are there some about which you are ambivalent? For example, "I am raised to have my family as a central part of my life and energies, but I am ambitious and want to focus on taking care of me. I am therefore pulled between them and me." Or "I am raised to value people getting along without much dissonance or discord. I then enter the medical world of academic sparring. On one hand, I feel I must be competitive so I can fit in. On the other

3

hand, I prefer to avoid conflict and am drained by being highly competitive."
We are pulled in both directions, one that we prefer and one we feel we should
follow.

Which do you prefer?

Working in a group	Working as a lone wolf
Connecting with others	Staying distant from others
Having harmonious relationships	Sparring relationships with others
Consensus is energizing	Debating or arguing is energizing
Being phony is offensive	Being phony is part of the game
Playing the game is draining	Playing the game is energizing
Time is relative	Punctuality is essential
Authority should be deferred to	Authority should be challenged
"Tooting your own horn" is immodest	"Tooting your own horn" is a savvy strategy
Being valued as "good" means being a hard worker	Being valued as "good" means being a quick study

Consider the preceding statements. Which do you prefer? Resist the temptation to say, "I value both equally," because this limits your ability to explore
which direction you tend to be pulled toward (especially when under stress.)
The exploration may help you anticipate personal challenges as you become
immersed in the medical culture.

Explore the role of your ethnic identity. Some of us have been raised to
value and cherish our cultures; others have been raised to deny or minimize
our differences. Regardless, how have you adapted to the stressors of not
appearing mainstream? Ask, What is internalized and ignored? What kind of
person do people see when they see me? It may seem odd to ask ourselves the
questions "How Black, Latino, Native American, am I?" "How Black, Latino,
Native American am I perceived?" "How comfortable am I with being Black,
Latino, Native American?" "What cultural influences and values have I
adopted as my own?" To enable the intentional creation of a physician identity where you can be comfortable, you need to understand yourself, to
include your values in the process. I suggest you use a tricultural approach—

evaluating your cultural world, that of majority culture, and that of medical culture. This will allow you the opportunity to determine what energizes and drains you, what you need to preserve, and what can be malleable as you enter the world of medicine (Núñez, 1992).

What Is This Place?

The world of medicine is exciting, filled with intellectual challenges, and life-and-death events. The practice of medicine gives us the opportunity to truly help our patients change their lives and lead healthier ones. The field is diverse enough that whatever your area of interest—analyzing the slide to diagnose disease, excising a diseased gallbladder, interpreting difficult symptoms to correctly treat illness, or counseling a patient to leave an abusive setting—medicine has a field suitable for you. As you go through your training, you will learn the dictionary, then the encyclopedia, of the language. You will learn about diseases and their causes and then begin acquiring and practicing the skills you will employ in the diagnosis and treatment of illness. Along the way, you will meet different groups of doctors—internists, pediatricians, surgeons, psychiatrists, family physicians, obstetrician/gynecologists—and you will learn about the unique parameters of each world. As you adapt to different settings and expectations, you will begin to understand the spectrum of the practice of medicine. Going through the process is a challenging experience.

In the United States in the early 1900s, medicine was primarily a world of White men. Historically, access to medical training for ethnic and religious minorities and for women was restricted (Lyons & Petrucelli, 1978). Schools would literally not allow certain people to apply. Slowly, the barriers lessened and underrepresented minorities gained some access to training. Because change was slow in coming, new schools such as the historically Black colleges were created to provide training opportunities (Curtis, 1971; Lyons & Petrucelli, 1978). A huge disparity still exists between the demographics of the population and of the physicians accepted into medical school today. Even if we are not the only persons of color around in our institutions, because of the continued disparities, we may still feel quite alone.

The Rules and Structure of the Medical World

So what are the traditions of the world of medicine (Christakis & Feudtner, 1993)? The structure and values of this system were formed by its initial membership but have evolved to reflect a more diverse medical culture. At times, it may be difficult to differentiate between mainstream culture and medical culture. These traditions are not inherently good or bad; they just are. Once you are able to see the overt and covert rules of this world, you can recognize how they fit with your values and traditions.

Often, the world of medicine is likened to a "game." "Playing the game" has nothing to do with goofing off. It means that you understand the system of the medical world and that you work within it. Playing the game implies that you follow the rules. The danger of this approach is that it may myopically convert the medical education process to a series of hoops you must jump through and totally miss the point of medical education—learning to think critically in a scientific way to solve problems and help patients. The advantage of the game analogy is that it can help us understand some of the underlying constructs of the medical world. There are a number of basic rules in medicine, and it is useful to understand where they came from, what they are, and how you can interact with this new culture most effectively. They center on hierarchy, power and influence, confidence and assertiveness, objectivity, task focus, giving 400%, and competition. Table 1.1 summarizes valuable information about understanding and interpreting medical rules.

Rule 1: Hierarchy

The medical world is hierarchical. The first rule is to *observe the hierarchy*. Power and responsibility are not shared equally. Success is rewarded in quantitative ways, such as the logbooks created to demonstrate proficiency in procedures. Competition is valued. Success results in promotion ("moving up the ladder"), and those higher up are compensated better than those on the lower rungs. People know where they stand. Individuals can gain recognition through excellence or even earn the right to respectfully challenge the leader.

The simplest hierarchical medical team is that of a learner and a senior practitioner. More complicated and formal are the hierarchies of the inpatient work teams in which a senior or attending physician supervises senior residents, who in turn supervise interns, who supervise students. In this hierarchy, "orders" are given with the intention of having others carry them out. Completion of these tasks is considered the goal. An interesting dynamic occurs in the medical setting. If you work well with others and do everything you are told, you can either be rewarded for being a good member of the team or, by contrast, be punished for not showing enough initiative or enthusiasm. Thus, in medical training, you will have to learn how to balance the expectations of being a good team member while distinguishing yourself among your peers.

Table 1.1 Understanding and Interpreting Medical Rules

Rule	Rationale	How It Might Feel	Potential Problems	Benefit to the Team
Hierarchy: The power structure flows from a chief downward through many layers of minions.	Lines of reporting are clear and consistent.	I am at the bottom of a large and oppressive pile.	Bullies may emerge, especially in systems in which there are long hours and rigorous schedules. The abused may be allowed to be abusers of people below them in the system to vent frustration and anger.	Members at the bottom benefit from the knowledge and experience of those at the top.
	Respect is afforded those at the top because of their prior contributions.	I get no respect because I haven't had time to contribute (my self-worth comes into question.)		Members at the top benefit from the time and efforts of those at the bottom.
	Medicine is an apprenticeship system.	The educational focus is not on me; it is on getting the work done.		Even negative role models can be useful to help people examine several styles.
Time: Everybody must be on time for rounds.	Work needs to get done in an efficient fashion.	Bowing to someone else's rules is demeaning (rules for the sake of rules).	The unpredictability of clinical medicine may make it difficult for you to adhere to a standard schedule. (Being late runs the risk of getting negatively labeled.)	Being on time shows respect for other members of the team's time.
	Structuring of time improves flow.	Often, lower-rung members have to wait for superiors.		Being on time demonstrates acceptance of the goal of getting the work done efficiently.
Interpersonal relations: Teams are transient, and your specific personality and experiences have no place.	Teams change frequently. The bottom of the hierarchy is large compared with the top.	You are an insignificant cog in a very large machine.	The team may miss out on the valuable experiences and knowledge of members of the team lower in the hierarchy.	Appropriate team members' self-care includes not investing too much emotional energy on transient members of the team.

(continued)

Table 1.1 Continued

Rule	Rationale	How It Might Feel	Potential Problems	Benefit to the Team
Scientific objectivity is a key component of interpersonal relationships. In **educational interactions**, it is assumed that the attending knows how and what to teach the members of the team.	The limited time available can be spent on the "business" of taking care of patients and educating members of the team rather than attending to personal matters.	Nothing of who you are counts. The system is cruel and unfeeling. Your needs (especially your learning needs) don't count.	Opportunities for empathy are missed. Individual learning styles may be neglected in favor of the learning style of the majority of the team members.	Work gets done in an expeditious manner. Dysfunctional teams are only temporary. Your learning is based on a standard rather than on an individualized program that may interfere with your learning the appropriate breadth of knowledge.
Self-promotion: There is a fine line between appropriate assertiveness and being overly aggressive.	With limited time exposure, attendings can know only what you demonstrate to them on rounds.	You are being pressured to perform in front of your peers, potentially making you feel like a fool. The others on your team will not like you if you are either incompetent or viewed as trying to make them look incompetent.	People with reserved personalities get read as not knowing/lacking knowledge. People with outgoing personalities get read as being "gunners."	Information can be shared quickly and efficiently when team members speak up and create opportunities for discussion/debate of key points.

SOURCE: Núñez and Webb (1995-1998).

Unfortunately, misperceptions on your part or by others can create difficulties (Christakis & Feudtner, 1993). If I express my enthusiasm by being very passionate or forceful, I may be misread as overly emotional or not sufficiently objective or dispassionate. If I misinterpret brusque, task-focused communications to be insensitive to me as a person rather than attending to the primary goal of patient care, I feel slighted or offended. Your ability to balance expectations and adapt to changing situations are key skills you will need to acquire for a successful career in medicine.

Although times are changing slowly, men are more often socialized to the hierarchical model, whereas women are socialized to a more collaborative style (Helgeson, 1990, 1996). The collaborative style is more democratic. It favors working toward consensus and collaboration over "winning" (Hall, 1994). Whether you were raised in a hierarchical or collaborative model, you can certainly function in either system. How well you function, how energizing or depleting these systems are depends on your personal preferences and on recognizing the advantages of both systems.

Rule 2: Power and Influence

Whether recognized overtly or covertly, doctors have *power and influence. You must manage yours appropriately.* Doctors have power over patients. Patients are sick and we are well. Patients come to our world, a foreign land of jargon and instruments and procedures. We know the language and have the tools. And despite shifting public opinion about physicians of late, doctors, for the most part, are still held in high regard. You will have ample opportunities to watch many physicians' styles as they deal with power and influence. On one end of the continuum, some physicians take the attitude that patients need to "follow directions" and do as they are told in order to get well. This doctoring style is considered high control, where the physician holds the power and expects compliance. On the other end of the continuum, doctors develop a more collaborative, low-control style with patients. They ask patients what they might do and negotiate for common goals. Long term, the patient will more likely follow the jointly decided plan rather than the mandated plan. Thus, low-control styles may result in more optimal health outcomes. Some doctoring styles you will choose to emulate; others, which may be abusive in their use of power, you may choose to reject.

The rule is very evident during training. Medical schools are similar to military academies. They all train people to "earn their stripes," to undergo certain rites of passage, and to assume their role in the system. There are some that rationalize the hardships of sleep deprivation and verbally abusive intellectual testing as simply the costs of joining the world of medicine. Although you do need to be strong enough to handle life-and-death challenges, occasionally these hardships are perpetuated because the physician has the attitude "I had to do it, so you will too." During your training, you have an opportunity to intentionally improve the system by not perpetuating the abuse.

Rule 3: Confidence and Assertiveness

The academic style in medicine is that of confrontational learning. This differs from other cultures in which learned professors bestow knowledge and challenging the authority is considered disrespectful. U.S. medicine encourages the learner to ask questions, even (within limits) questioning authority and insisting on being heard (Bloom, 1988). Another rule, then, is that *participants must exhibit confidence and assertiveness.* This often manifests in the clinical years, while on junior clerkships, as roundsmanship. *Roundsmanship* is the term used for the educational interaction that occurs while you round on hospitalized patients on your service. The attending often asks difficult questions related to the patients in a rapid-fire manner, trying to stump the students and residents. Keeping up with the academic sparring, being sufficiently extroverted to participate, and being able to handle the frequently blunt retorts if you answer incorrectly are all important confidence and assertiveness skills you will need. A number of years ago, an article in the lay press described a new syndrome, perhaps most aptly titled the "Always Being Right Syndrome" (Campbell, 1992). This syndrome was described, tongue-in-cheek, as an illness in which individuals felt the need to (a) always provide an answer, (b) always convey their opinions in a fashion that was convincing and resolute (regardless of whether they were correct), and (c) challenge anyone who questioned them. Too often, this syndrome afflicts our field. This may, in part, be an issue of ego or trust. That is, "If you don't think I can answer all your questions, how can you trust me?" Thus, credibility becomes blurred with "always being right" or always having an answer. The responsibility for this tendency does not lie only on the physician's doorstep. Too often, patients expect us to be human ATM machines. Ask a question, get an instant answer. The "Always Being Right" Answer Syndrome often has students answer loudly and proudly even if they do not have the right answer. For many people, this presents an enormous challenge. How can I present myself confidently when I am unsure? If I act in this way, am I not being cocky? Phony? If I overstep and am caught misrepresenting information, won't I be viewed as being untrustworthy? Fundamentally, all humans, including doctors, are fallible. The practice of medicine, much as we wish it to be different, includes errors. Our pledge is to do no intentional harm, and to learn from our errors. We all learn from our successes, but more often, we learn even more from our mistakes. If you knew all that you needed to know to be a doctor, you would not have to go through the process.

Being a "fast study," a student who quickly catches on and appears to do this in an effortless fashion, is valued in medicine. You will find areas in medicine that come to you quickly and other areas that cause you to struggle. Realize that the "fast study" is often a created image, not reality. Too often, students believe a colleague who brags about not studying for important examinations. There are far more students who present themselves as brilliant than the actual number of brilliant students who effortlessly learn medicine. Do not be lured into following in their purported footsteps because this will be a recipe for academic disaster!

Finally, there is a fine line between assertive behavior versus aggressive behavior. Assertiveness that challenges and acknowledges the hierarchy is rewarded. If I question a plan of treatment because I have read of another effective treatment, I am likely to be rewarded for my initiative. If I ask for feedback on my clinical performance and ask to meet my attending at a time that suits their schedule, I am being assertive and respectful. Aggressiveness is overstepping the line. If I question *every* treatment plan, I may be judged as too difficult to work with, insubordinate, or at the least, not being "a team player." If I demand feedback on my clinical performance now, I am being aggressive and disrespectful. Being perceived as assertive rather than aggressive can be challenging. If you feel deeply about a situation, your emotional overtones can be misread as aggressive, even if you do not mean to send this message.

Rule 4: Scientific Objectivity

Objectivity in medicine is the gold standard. This implies that we are able to view situations in totally unemotional, dispassionate ways. One reason for this cultural goal is that objectivity should help you gain a clear picture of the issues you need to address. Another reason is that in medical culture, emotions are to be feared. They are, by definition, not logical and not readily controlled. They flavor our perspective and have us react from the heart, not the head. This fear of emotion is evident in physicians' reluctance or aversion toward emotionally challenging tasks—that is, breaking bad news and obtaining information about end-of-life choices. A third reason for this cultural goal is that objectivity creates a distance between the patient and us. This distance protects us and enables us to perform tasks that would be impossible if we felt them ourselves. For example, if you personally envisioned the pain caused from a needle inserted into the spine for a lumbar puncture (spinal tap), you might not be able to perform a life-saving procedure and accurately diagnose meningitis. Objectivity helps us define "me" versus "not me." There is merit in being able to balance emotion with logic; at the same time, it is unlikely that we can "rid" ourselves of our emotional lenses. Therefore, if you are someone who is in tune with others' feelings, the system may feel cruel and unfeeling. To succeed, you may need to work toward acquiring a task-focused, logical approach to balance your style. If you are already task focused, you may need to work on understanding the impact of illness on your patients and on enhancing your empathic skills.

Rule 5: Task Focused Over Interpersonal Focused

Another rule in medicine is to focus on "getting the job done." There is *heavy emphasis on being task focused,* not focused on the impact of the disease or on the interpersonal relationships involved. This rule fits well with that of objectivity. If all we see is the problem, then our task is solving it. It also skirts around interpersonal and emotional challenges, which are less efficiently "fixed."

Many of you will be taught, during your "preclinical" or "basic science years," to take time with your patients, to develop skills in addressing the impact of illness on the patients' lives. The task-focused concentration during the clinical years may seem contrary to this teaching. Sick patients enter the hospital and are expected to leave in a short period of time with all their needs addressed. The time constraints of getting patients in and out of the hospital quickly translate into the task focus of medicine. We have a lot to do: orders to put in, tests to run, consults to obtain, and of course, very little time. The attending, with the resident's input, establishes a plan; the intern, with the resident's oversight, implements the plan. The students help to complete the plan.

However, for effective care, we all need to be expert in the interpersonal impact of illness with our patients. We often have too few role models to show us. This is not necessarily because people do not care. Rather, it is probably a combination of feeling uncomfortable and feeling pressured for time. Connecting with patients and effectively eliciting their feelings in a supportive but manageable way is not as easy a skill as doing a procedure or evaluating a lab result. Often in training, it is glossed over. Make a special effort to seek out physicians who model these abilities and watch closely how they work with their patients. We are in an era in which physicians are responsible to be "smart" and make the right diagnosis and also to ensure optimal health outcomes of their patients. The skill of interpersonal effectiveness becomes an essential one.

Rule 6: Giving 400%

The expectation in medicine is that *individuals must give 400%* in terms of time, energy, and interest. This is interpreted as being truly devoted to your tasks and being serious about your work. Some continue to hold the conviction that unless you can "run the code while sleep deprived" or deliver care correctly despite lack of food and sleep, you are not a good doctor. No request, then, is unreasonable. Failure to give superhuman performance is interpreted as lack of motivation, ability, or interest. Medicine is not a field in which you can dabble. It takes mental and physical stamina to stay the course.

Rule 7: The "Game"—Academic Competition

To be recognized as a legitimate member of the team, *you must "play the game."* This aspect of working within the system means engaging in the academic sparring in a competitive setting. Participating is not enough. You must demonstrate your intellectual prowess at problem solving, usually tested by verbally presented challenges that you must solve on the spot. This competition may be perceived as heartless. A correct answer is meagerly rewarded. An incorrect answer may generate a snide or insulting response. (The reality, however, is that students are expected to make mistakes. Knowing when you are in over your head and asking for help is an important skill.)

Playing the game and believing that you must always have the right answer is not realistic or humane. For most students, it is better to reframe the game, from always being correct to always trying, contributing in conference or rounds, putting yourself "out there." The students who focus on trying their best are able to endure the game better than those who put superhuman expectations on themselves. Some students are intimidated by the game and are frequently silent, in fear of being wrong. The reality is that quiet students are judged as lacking knowledge or as apathetic. Students who risk answering and who can tolerate criticism are viewed as smart, enthusiastic, and tough enough. Perhaps one of the most challenging and frustrating aspects of the game is that there is more than one. The expectations and etiquette of a surgery clerkship during your third year are very different from those of your psychiatry clerkship, which are different from your medicine clerkship. For example, if you wanted to talk to "the person in charge" in surgery, you most likely would speak to your senior resident or the chief surgical resident. In medicine, more likely you would speak to the attending physician. The nature of rounds and your function on the team varies from discipline to discipline. The advantage of seeing many types of teams is that you will likely find the one that suits you and that will be the direction of your career. To succeed, you need to analyze expectations, convey your abilities to others, and take care of yourself in every rotation you take.

Taking My Place Within the Culture of Medicine

Verbal Expression

As mentioned before, the verbal interactions that occur in medicine consist of succinct bits of data delivered rapidly in a proscribed style. A patient's case is presented as such: "Ms. Jones is a 42-year-old woman with a history of insulin-dependent diabetes who presents with shortness of breath." Questions regarding the case are often interjected during the presentation, which can cause the student to lose track of the story as he or she presents the case. During typical "rounds," the attending or chief physician will ask rapid-fire questions about the diseases the patients have. The purpose of the questions is to elicit the student's fund of knowledge on illness and treatment options. Long-winded presentations are not tolerated and are cut off. This communication style relies heavily on verbal abilities and extroversion. Be succinct and convey information quickly. Learn to tolerate interruptions, respond to questions, and return to the presentation. Additionally, you must handle blunt and occasionally abusive criticism without becoming emotional.

This Morse code type of communication—short bursts of information and data—is different from other types of communication. Compare this with two other communication styles, that of the minister at the pulpit and that of the storyteller.

The communication style of the Black minister at the pulpit is successful in the appropriate setting: The goal of the communication is to connect with the audience emotionally. Establishing the connection is as important as the message or the point. Being able to feel the communication, not just understand the idea, is important. The facts, of course, are important. But understanding the message means being able to send it on an emotional level.

Now consider the style of the storyteller. Storytellers rely on painting a visual image of the situation. They use words, like paint, to create a scene and set up the story. Messages are conveyed indirectly and with subtlety. The storyteller sets the stage, paints the picture, and invites the audience to participate in the process of the story. The experience is as important as the point of the message.

In the medical style of communication described above, the emotional impact is irrelevant or, at least, should be purged from delivering the data. It does not include "experiencing the story." The only focus is the data. If you use a style similar to that of the minister, you could be misread as overly verbose or angry. If you use the storyteller style, you could be misread as unfocused or overly familiar. Both styles fail to conform to medical standards. Using these styles puts you at risk for being misjudged. You may be viewed as lacking knowledge (the key facts about their patients) even if you know the important data—all because you did not present quickly or concisely.

Strive to add to your repertoire a modification of your verbal (and written) delivery style that conforms to the standard. Do you tend to talk a while to get the point? Are you very enthusiastic and sometimes misread as overbearing? Is it difficult for you to put yourself out in front? Usually, you get a few minutes a day to convey your knowledge and talents to faculty members who are evaluating you. Get feedback from others, especially from trusted mentors, to modify your delivery style and send the message you want.

Being able to read your audience ("Hmm, this is the attending who likes the one-minute presentation versus the one who likes the ten-minute presentation") is also important. Each team you work with differs. The members' personalities blend to create a group temperament. Watch and listen carefully to the way that the senior team members present and write their notes so that you can uncover unspoken expectations. Seek feedback from residents or faculty members on how to adjust your style and your written communication. This flexibility is absolutely key in presenting the information you know in a way that will be well received. It is an essential skill for you to get appropriate credit for your abilities.

Time

In medicine, there never seems to be enough time. Even during the preclinical years, students feel the pressure. If you read every assigned reading given, training would have to be extended by years! Hospitals are geared to rapid admissions and discharges. Students who are just beginning their training find in-patient activity chaotic and confusing. The outpatient setting is not any more leisurely. With large volumes of patients waiting in crowded waiting rooms, students are pressured into rapidly finding out what is "wrong" and what the patient "wants." Residents are stressed in trying to get patients "out." Faculty members juggle multiple commitments to teach, to deliver care, and to be academically productive (Mechanic, 1991).

This perspective of time as a scarce resource manifests itself in the language of medicine. We use jargon and abbreviations. Often, telephone conversations sound more like Morse code than actual discourse. We become used to deleting the social niceties: "Hello." and "How are you?" are reduced to a "What?" This stress spills into patient care and can manifest as impatience, distraction, and even anger. Patients who make our lives easy get rewarded. Those who do not get labeled as "difficult patients."

Sometimes, the pressure of time constraints is real. You cannot wait to run a code on a patient with a dropping blood pressure. Sometimes, the pressure is self-imposed. Rushing about can be energizing. Sometimes we forget and rush as a habit versus as a necessity. Time constraints may make us rush about for a number of reasons beyond habit. We may very well have too many responsibilities, or rushing may help us feel that we are doing important work. We may not be taking sufficient care of our personal lives and are at risk of burnout. It is useful to try to recognize and triage the different immediacies in our lives to avoid being swept away with the moment.

One of the requirements in medicine, at least for those lower on the ladder, is being on time. For good evaluations, be early, if not exactly on time. Under *no* circumstances allow stereotypes, such as "minorities are never on time," to be attributed to your actions. Although you cannot control the opinions of others, you can prevent opportunities to mislabel your behavior. Always be on time!

Conclusion

Remember, you have been selected as the "cream of the crop." You deserve to be here—in medical school. You may be able to understand patients that many of your classmates can not. Your contributions to caring for patients will enable our profession to achieve the goal of appropriate and effective care for all patients. Developing the flexibility of "fitting into the system" may seem like a sellout. But that is true only if you forget who you are in the process. Only those who succeed in the system can create meaningful change. Do well and succeed. Work together to make the process and the profession more balanced and caring as you do the same in your own lives.

Sample Conflicts

Below are some examples of student challenges or conflicts. Consider each of the scenarios below. How might you act in each setting? How easy or difficult would it be to actually do what is recommended in the resolution, based on your personality?

Scenario 1   You need to study material, and it is not coming easily. You do not want to ask the lecturer questions for several reasons: You were raised to be respectful to authority, including professors; you are reluctant to "bother them with a stupid question"; and it seems like "brownnosing." You notice that other students are not shy about talking to the professor. It seems to you that they are just trying to brownnose. You spend hours by yourself trying to figure it out (instead of hours covering important material on the test.) Your classmates do far better than you on the exam. They go up to the professor and ask questions all the time.

Resolution: Recognize that the greater goal (academic success) makes you violate the cultural norm of questioning authority, and force yourself to go talk to professors.

Scenario 2   You are more comfortable working in a group and not sticking out. On rounds you prefer not to jump in and appear rude. Other classmates jump in and talk a lot on ward rounds. Your evaluation returns as: "quiet, unsure of fund of knowledge, and unclear if interested in this field."

Resolution: Acknowledge that the rules of the clinical setting require you to put yourself forward, be more extroverted than you prefer. Work hard to demonstrate your abilities on rounds (see Chapter 5).

<u>Scenario 3</u>   You are comfortable with and enjoy talking. Your superiors, who never let you get to the point, put you off balance by constant interruptions. They cut you off all the time.

Resolution: Seek out your resident or faculty adviser and ask for help to improve the succinctness of your presentation. Practice at home with others to "get to the point" quickly. Strive to get out the sound bites that allow you to finish the story.

<u>Scenario 4</u>   You are assertive and outgoing. As you imitate the behavior of others on the team, you are pulled aside and told to be "less angry." You are confused by this comment.

Resolution: Consider that your energetic presentation may be misread as overly emotional and "angry." Despite what may seem unfair at this misread, recognize that your manner evokes an emotional response in others that will have negative consequences. Work on being more emotionally reserved in your presentations. Ask for help and feedback to be more accurately perceived (see Chapter 5).

<u>Scenario 5</u>   You face challenges in your studies and decide you are just not working hard enough. You increase your efforts and now

get three to four hours of sleep a night. You are irritable and stressed and still not doing well.

Resolution: "Harder" and "more" are not always better. It is important to reach out to course or clerkship directors, minority faculty advisers, and support people to change your focus. You may be working plenty hard, but you are not focused in the direction you need. Only if you get outside help will you be able to gain perspective and learn how to work differently, not just harder.

Scenario 6   You find that spending time with family and engaging in extracurricular activities energizes you. You have been raised to believe that family always comes first, and you value your family. As you become more stressed, you spend more time on nonschool activities. Finally, you find that you are far behind.

Resolution: Just as you need to expand your armamentarium of stress-reducing activities and support people, you need to work on balance. Family members can certainly provide support, but at times, they can also distract or drain your energy reserves. Avoid solving this challenge on your own. You may benefit from talking to a student services counselor, faculty member, or family member to help you understand what is disrupting your studies (see Chapter 7).

Scenario 7   You feel like you are being singled out and picked on by a faculty member. You become increasingly irritated with this person's behavior. You start coming to rounds late. Your evaluation reads, "poor attitude and work habits."

Resolution: Seek input from your resident on this issue. Meet with the faculty member and ask for his or her help in understanding what you need to do to improve your performance. Consider informing the clerkship director that there is a conflict you are working on trying to resolve (see Chapters 3 and 5).

Scenario 8   You are a junior clerk in a hospital with non-English-speaking environmental service workers. You are friendly and warm, greeting them every day in their language. The residents you work with begin to harass you, mocking the support services people. They say, "So, you like them better than us?"

Resolution: Remember, you work as a member of a team. Some teams have stronger rules of conformity and belonging. In these teams, you are either "with us" or "against us." Identification with others can put you at risk for abuse. Your ability to speak a language other than English, because it excludes others (especially those in the hierarchy who are supposed to have power over you) makes others uncomfortable and nervous. This polar view of the world, "with us" or "against us," can be draining. You can choose to interact less with hospital workers or you can choose to challenge your residents on their harassing behavior. Which you select depends on your personality. Remember that harassment, specifically sexual harassment, should be reported to an attending, the clerkship director, or the dean.

REFERENCES

Bloom, S. (1988). Structure and ideology in medical education: An analysis of resistance to change. *Journal of Health and Social Behavior, 29,* 294-306.

Campbell, J. (1992, January/February). Male answer syndrome. *Utne Reader,* pp. 107-108.

Christakis, D., & Feudtner, C. (1993). Ethics in a short white coat: The ethical dilemmas that medical students confront. *Academic Medicine, 68,* 249-254.

Curtis, J. (1971). *Blacks, medical schools, and society.* Ann Arbor: University of Michigan Press.

Hall, J. (1994). Gender in medical encounters: An analysis of physician and patient communication in a primary care setting. *Health Psychology, 13,* 384-392.

Helgeson, S. (1990). *The female advantage: Women's ways of leadership.* New York: Doubleday.

Helgeson, S. (1996). *The web of inclusion: Building an organization for everyone.* New York: Doubleday.

Lyons, A., & Petrucelli, J. (1978). *Medicine: An illustrated history.* New York: Harry N. Abrams.

Mechanic, D. (1991). Sources of countervailing power in medicine. *Journal of Health Political Policy and Law, 16,* 485-498.

Núñez A. (1992). *Looking within to see the outside better: A course in cultural diversity and medicine. Internal medicine* [internally published]. Philadelphia, PA: MCP Hahnemann University. (Available from the author)

Núñez, A., & Webb, C. (1995-1998). *Navigating the medical culture: Medical student course curricular document* [internally published] (4th ed.). Philadelphia, PA: MCP Hahnemann University. (Available from the authors)

2 Mastering the First Two Years

CARMEN WEBB, MD
MORRIS HAWKINS, JR., PHD

From the first day of orientation, you become immersed in the medical culture we've described in Chapter 1. Some things are very similar to college or postbaccalaureate programs: You amass and digest information through didactic or self-directed learning; you take countless exams. It's when you see the amount of material you are expected to learn, the level of detail, the long class hours—not to speak of the personal adjustment to this very new world— that you feel the real difference. Both the academic task and the personal task are necessary; they lay the foundation for the rest of your journey through medicine. This chapter is designed to address some of the academic and personal challenges you will face in dealing with these tasks and to offer specific suggestions for managing them effectively.

Preparing Yourself

Prematriculation Programs

As you prepare to start medical school, you may feel you've got a pretty solid idea of what the experience will be like. Possibly you have attended a premed orientation, gone to a Medical Student Zero (premed) weekend, or shadowed a physician. Yet as valuable as these opportunities are, they don't replace prematriculation programs as windows to the medical school world. Many majority schools have such summer programs for accepted minority students. Some may even be offered to students as a condition of acceptance (Shields, 1994). So if you're invited, go! There, you will be introduced to medical culture. You will have an opportunity to get comfortable with your level of preparedness (because you will likely sample some course work) rather than to blindly accept the myths about all minorities "not being ready" for medical school. What many students remember most about these programs is the opportunity to build relationships and unity ("we're in this together") with other minorities. The whole experience can make your transition into first year much easier.

Orientation

Usually, the first formal activity in medical school for all students is orientation. You will be inundated with "get-acquainted" activities and with welcoming speeches, from everyone from the dean to the parking garage manager. This first week can be lots of fun, however, when you begin to receive stacks of materials, books, and syllabi. And as you realize how much is really going to be covered, these days can also be overwhelming and a little scary. Some students choose to skip the orientation activities that are not required, either by being physically absent or by mentally/emotionally zoning out. Try very hard to be present during this time. You will not be able to retain all the information offered, but at least you will have it filed somewhere. More important, you will have an opportunity to get a feel of the culture of your medical school and to form alliances with many of your classmates. This is the time people are most open to new relationships.

If you are one of those students accepted late in the summer and therefore miss orientation, make a point to go to Student Affairs and ask to receive all the materials distributed during that week.

In the Classroom

During the first two years, you spend substantial time in the classroom, sometimes from 8 or 9 a.m. to 4 or 5 p.m. Although it is possible to spend your whole day in the same large lecture hall, in 50-minute classes and with 10- to 15-minute breaks, your schedule will include small-group learning and occasional patient contact. Your lecture attendance is voluntary. The exams are not. Make a point to discern early the impact of your class attendance on your learning and performance.

At most schools, you learn about normal body function the first year. Some of your course work may be done on a computer, and you may be required to have on computer on admission. In the second year, you'll cover abnormal body function—disease and treatment. You usually have clinical exposure by the second semester of the second year (conducting histories and physical exams with patients). It's exciting to finally be starting the business of doctoring and applying all your newly acquired knowledge to patients.

> "I started out confident about Biochemistry since I'd had it the year before, as a premed. But then we covered in one week what I'd learned in an entire quarter in college."

During these two years, the volume of information you are assigned is nothing short of incredible (and awfully close to ridiculous) (Committee on Education Group, 1982). Despite some lore to the contrary, the amount of material is not assigned to "weed people out." The fact is, the intricacies of the human body and the level of detail therein are also incredible. So the work in medical school is necessarily immense.

In the Labs

You will be responsible for laboratory classes to help you to apply classroom knowledge. Labs can clarify concepts and have tremendous application to "real-life medicine." In some cases, you'll be able to choose your lab partners. Think this choice through carefully. Often, the option is given at the beginning of the year when you don't know people well. Students tend to choose whomever they are friendly with at the time. Minority students in a majority school may gravitate toward one another. Comfort with the people you work with in such close proximity is extremely important. This may indeed be the best option for you, but be sure you are not overlooking important issues—such as whether or not you have similar work styles (you may have learned this in your prematriculation program). If your group is all minority in a majority school, find a way to obtain resources that majority students may be passing around (like a great new anatomy atlas that a fourth-year recommended). Know also that your cadre will be under particular scrutiny: Unfortunately, individuals in all-minority groups will very often be expected to perform similarly, and the entire group may not be expected to perform as well as other groups.

Depending on your learning style (or your stamina), you may be tempted to skip labs altogether or to come in to the lab outside of class time. Even if this strategy works well for you, be careful. If your physical characteristics readily identify you as a minority student (especially in a majority school), the professor will note your absence. You may not hear about it immediately, but if you have any difficulty in the course, your professors will likely comment, "well he never came to lab," translated "he was disinterested, lazy, didn't try and/or deserves to receive the low grade/to remediate." A majority student may certainly be evaluated similarly, *if* the professors notice he or she is gone.

Anatomy Lab

In anatomy lab, you and three to five lab partners will be responsible for dissecting and learning about one part of the human body at a time. Lab instructors will be available to help you find structures and to understand what you see. And because all human bodies are different, you learn a lot from computer software and from looking at the cadavers of other groups. Sometimes the lab instructor will wander over to your table and begin to ask questions. "What is the name of this structure?" "What nerve enervates this muscle?" Whether the questioning is formal (graded) or informal, this may be your first introduction to the Socratic teaching method employed by most medical schools (see Chapter 3). When your group is questioned, remember that the language of medical culture applies: be brief, succinct, assertive, and confident in your answers. If a question is given to the whole table and you know—or think you know—the answer, speak up. If you are wrong, you are wrong. But if you say nothing, the instructor will assume that you *know* nothing. Even if you aren't graded, consider the experience practice for "quizzing" on the wards (Fine, 1994) (see Chapters 1 and 3).

The Cadaver

For almost all medical students, the cadaver brings up many feelings. If you have experienced the death of someone close to you or a death that affected you strongly, you may be surprised by a rush of feelings before, during, or after working on your cadaver. If you are concerned about your own health or death, the body may scare you (Kaplan & Sadock, 1989, p. 1343). The idea of cutting a human may feel disrespectful. Or you may just experience anger and anxiety, without knowing the source. Fortunately, many schools recognize the stress of this experience and have mechanisms (e.g., orientation, memorial services, and small-group discussions) to help students deal with their reactions. If this help is not enough, talk things out with a counselor. The worst thing to do is to adopt an armor that hides your real feelings (even from yourself). Dealing with reactions now will help you manage your feelings toward your dying patients later on (Kaplan & Sadock, 1989).

Some cultures have views of death and of dead bodies that are significantly different from those of mainstream America. Depending on your background, you may have very specific concerns not understood by your professors and peers from different cultures (Galanti, 1991).

> One African American student noted that she and her family believe that the spirit of the dead is very much present and watching over the living. To dissect a body was a desecration and a dishonor to the dead.

If you have cultural concerns or conflicts such as these, consult with your course director. Be ready to clearly explain your views and to suggest options (e.g., I will come to lab and watch, but not participate in the dissection). If your views are not respected, decide how strongly you feel about the situation and consider carefully if this is a request to bring to the dean of student affairs, minority affairs, or academic affairs.

What If My Way Doesn't Work Anymore?

Top students enter medical school every year expecting to maintain the same study habits they used in the past. In college, you may have found that if you would just read and memorize all the material assigned, you could do well on the exams. Now, in medical school, you are doing the same things, but for some reason, you can never cover all the material. Your grades have begun to suffer. Although you will almost certainly be studying more than you ever have, the reality is that mastery is impossible (see the "Balance" section later in this chapter,) and integration of the material must accompany memorization. Bottom line: The trusted method that got you here may not work anymore. To decide if you need a new approach, stop and do an academic self-assessment.

Let's say that you get your grades from your first set of exams and you are not pleased.

1. *First: Review your approach to your academic work.* Do you attend lecture? How do you take notes? Do you use a study group? The computer lab?

Your exam schedule, your study schedule, and everything else that affects your academic work should be considered.

2. *Second: Question your approach.* Ask yourself, your adviser(s), faculty members, peers, and counselors to help you isolate any potential problems or areas of inefficiency. You need input from outside. What are the advantages or disadvantages of having a study schedule? Should you start attending (or skipping) certain classes? Are you scheduling enough (or too much) time for eating, sleeping, transportation, and the like? Even if you hate studying in groups, could that help? Do you need to answer test questions differently? What are some alternatives to the approach that will be more effective? Don't leave any area unexplored.

3. *Third: Begin to make changes.* It is extremely important that you make changes only after Steps 1 and 2. It is seldom beneficial to suddenly switch your habits, mimicking those of someone else who gets better grades, without knowing why. In addition, don't make changes all at once. If you do, you have no way of evaluating which changes are responsible for the progress you are making. Remember, you may have to reassess periodically for different courses. *Special Note: Make sure your change is not "I will only study and cut out all else." That approach is certain to fail. (Read on.)*

Be aware that changing your style may be a little frightening. You are giving up the trusted help that brought you here in exchange for the unknown. But trust your academic self-assessment.

Balance: How Is It Possible?

Your premed adviser probably insisted that you have to really work to make it in medical school and to give up a great deal if you want to succeed. On the other hand, no doubt people have cautioned you, "Make sure you take some time for fun." Great advice from both camps, but no one really tells you just *how,* with classes all day and studying in the evening, to fit both study and leisure time into your life. And that is what balance is: making time for both study and personal needs.

The Problem: Two Scenarios

Tomas was well aware that it takes long hours and hard work to do well in medical school. To make sure he had time to study, he did little for relaxation except talk to friends on the telephone occasionally. On rare occasions, his roommates were able to drag him out to a movie. As the semester wore on, his friends noticed that he was becoming increasingly irritable, anxious, and tense.

Cynthia got very good grades in college and took pride in a tutoring service she developed for foster children. In medical school, she was elected president of the student body, volunteered in the AIDS clinic, and was treasurer of the Student National Medical Association (SNMA). She did not do well on the first biochemistry test but concluded she could not always be at the top of the class. Two weeks before a major exam, Cynthia took over coordinating a major student event. She now has to repeat biochemistry over the summer.

Both these students (Webb & Núñez, 1995-1998) are struggling with a real dilemma of balance. You may struggle also.

Why is balance so difficult? Why does the time required for studying seem limitless? Very often, it is because we are aiming to *master* the material presented (Committee on Education Group, 1982). In high school and college, you may have been able to learn everything backward and forward. Now you do not have that kind of time. Even if you studied 24 hours a day, the sheer volume of material and the level of detail you will be asked to absorb makes mastery humanly impossible (Becker, Geer, Hughes, & Strauss, 1961; Committee on Education Group, 1982). Medicine changes daily, and every patient is different. As a physician, it will be impossible to care for your patients day and night and still have time to read all the journals, attend enough conferences, learn about all the new drugs, and keep up with the research in the area. However, being in control is something that medical students and physicians value highly. Our sense of mastery allows us to feel in control: "I know this, so I will do well on that test." Or "I will be able to manage any patient with that illness." We feel confident in ourselves because we can direct the outcome. Loss of mastery, on the other hand, is one of the greatest losses suffered by students and physicians (Stein, 1990). So great is the loss that many can never accept it. But if you don't acknowledge your own limits, you will continually feel frustrated, disappointed, and eventually helpless, angry, or depressed.

Another reason that balance is difficult is that you will tend (and in fact the culture of medicine encourages you) to try to approach life by "doing it all." But you can't. It is not humanly possible to master all the medical material, much less to do so while giving sufficient attention to family, romantic relationships, friendships, household responsibilities, eating, sleeping, and, oh yeah, to yourself. If you remain unconvinced, try an experiment. Write down the number of hours each of these areas needs ideally for maintenance every week. No doubt your total is far greater than the 168 hours human beings are allotted.

Balance is your ability to gauge time necessary for both study and personal goals, then to spend time required for both types of activities. You must constantly reevaluate your activities so that you achieve a healthy balance between academic and personal pursuits.

Signs of Imbalance

How do you know if your life is tipping out of balance? If you are not studying enough, the signs are obvious. Your stack of unread lecture notes gets thicker, you can't seem to keep up in class, and your grades drop. If you are studying too much, the signs may not be as clear. Perhaps you can't concentrate as you used to. You don't care as much about learning the material. Your loved ones tell you that all you talk about is medical school. You don't know about the major catastrophe that just rocked the world.

The Solution, or How Do I Avoid Losing the Balance Game?

Let's imagine that you've accepted that you have limits. You can't master everything, and you can't tend to every life area. Well if you can't do it all, then something will have to go. The trick is to figure out what that something is.

Unhealthy Solution: Sacrifice Yourself

The values of medical culture suggest that you "put medicine first, everything else second, and if something has to go, sacrifice your personal needs" (A. Núñez, personal communication, June 1998; Stein, 1990). That's what a really responsible and caring physician would do, right? So we push our-selves. In fact, we all have that in common in medicine—the ability to push ourselves relentlessly. Minority students who have been schooled in this country have learned to push themselves even harder than their majority col-leagues because they have encountered so many obstacles. So typically, when the work is coming fast and furious, you will be inclined to continuously put out and do little (or inadequate) replenishment. You pump physical, emo-tional, and mental energy into anatomy lab—getting no sunlight, smelling of formaldehyde, cramming facts into your brain, and interfacing with all the dif-ferent personalities and stresses of your anatomy partners. How much do you put back in? If you just sleep, you may overcome the physical exhaustion, but you won't renew the emotional energy you put out in tolerating your know-it-all lab partner. If you go straight home to work on biochemistry, your brain has no time to rest. If the extent of your balancing effort is vegetating in front of the TV—watching whatever is on at the moment, you are taking much-needed time off from studying, but you aren't yet taking time to recharge. For awhile, you can probably handle this OK. But over time, usually by Novem-ber, that lifestyle gets old. If you keep it up, you'll probably complete medical school, but you also may be like one of those suitcases left on the airport conveyor belt long after all the rest have been collected, battered and beaten up (A. Núñez, personal communication, June 1998).

Healthy Solution: Sacrifice the Nonessential

Obviously, studying is important to you. If you don't study, you will not be in medical school very long, so evaluate the study time you will need to learn "enough," (you won't have a feel for this until a week or more into the course). Then schedule that study time. Repeat: Schedule that study time (Webb & Núñez, 1995-1998). Even if written schedules make you urticarial, keep a schedule in your head—a real schedule. (Recognize that it is easy to dupe yourself into fudging your time if you do not write the schedule down.) Then follow the sage advice of one minority affairs director: "Never steal time; borrow it. Then pay it back." If a free concert comes up the

> Balance requires three steps:
> ▶ Decide what/who is important to keep you growing physically, emo-tionally, mentally, and spiritually.
> ▶ Make time for those activities, people, or rest periods.
> ▶ Eliminate something that may be desirable but that is really not essential to keep you growing.

night you planned to review genetics, go only if you can decide *specifically* when you will make up that study time.

Deciding what recharges you is absolutely essential (Myers, 1998; Webb & Núñez, 1995-1998) (see Chapter 6). For now, consider, What is energizing to you? What is draining? What do you need? Once you have determined your needs for recharging, you will need to *set time aside specifically* for these things just as you did for studying. Think of it this way. Besides study time, which is a given, there is life maintenance time, time with others, and individual relaxation time.

- *Life maintenance time* may include time spent paying bills, going grocery shopping, cleaning up.
- *Time with others* means time spent with others that is important to maintain relationships.
- *Individual relaxation time* means spending time doing things that charge your engine. It does not count unless it truly gives you pleasure or fulfillment. Life maintenance time and time with others do *not* count toward individual relaxation time.

First, schedule individual relaxation time that belongs to you alone, every single day. It does not belong to family, friends, or kids. Start with a minimum amount of time and work your way up. Example: ½ to 1 hour per day on weekdays and 1 to 2 hours per day on the weekend. This may seem like an incredibly skimpy amount of time, but many students have a hard time finding it. When you prioritize, the place to trim is *not* individual relaxation time. You probably can trim some time off the other things within nonstudy time (let the dishes sit).

You will also need to schedule time with others, or it probably won't happen. It's much easier to put off getting together with others until "things lighten up." But in medical school, a "light period" is rare. You are not likely to get around to catching many movies with your spouse unless you specifically schedule them.

That is really the key. Schedule the time with significant people. If you are in a committed relationship with someone close by, schedule one date a week. It may just be a three- or four-hour period that you spend together at home with popcorn and music. The most important element of a date is for *you* to be fully present—not falling asleep, not complaining about your classmates, not reminding the other person of how much work you are putting on hold just to be with him or her. Talk together about how you would most like to spend the time. (The challenge here may be for you to listen to your significant other; you are self-absorbed now and likely to miss what your loved one is saying.) If you have a boyfriend or girlfriend in another city or if you have extended family members who haven't seen you in awhile, you may feel like you can't afford to spend the little free time you have with other friends. But because most students need to have friends among classmates as well, you probably want to schedule playtime with them at least once a month or so.

If you have children, you know that they are less likely to fall easily into a schedule. Keep a mental note of what will go if you need to drop things to tend to their needs. For instance, if you had planned to clean the bathroom, study physiology notes, and call an old friend one evening, but Little José gets sick, you can't physically get it all in. What needs to go? Probably the bathroom, but maybe it will be the old friend as well. If physiology goes, be sure to schedule it somewhere else.

Bottom line: There is much to do. And if you don't schedule time to recharge your battery, none of it will get done.

How Do I Not Feel Guilty
for Relaxation Time?

If you can't quite accept that "taking care of yourself" is a legitimate priority, recognize that without relaxation time to recharge your engine, you will not be able to study effectively for the long haul (Webb & Núñez, 1995-1998). No matter what you've endured in the past, your new identity of "medical student" puts you in a high-risk group for anxiety, depression, marital difficulties, and more. If you don't recharge, you will likely become a statistic. If that's still not enough to assuage your guilt, recognize that without time off, your stress will leak out somewhere, and it will probably be onto those closest to you. (You'll start behaving like the self-absorbed physician that you swore you'd never be!)

Summary

As a student, and later as a physician, the healthiest goal is to acknowledge your limits. Accept your loss of mastery and work toward a standard of excellence that is *attainable*. Identify the essential parts that keep you going. Sacrifice the nonessential.

Managing Competition

From the day you hear the statistics about the number of applications versus acceptances to medical school, you are warned of the competitive nature of your pursuit. You may wonder how you will stack up next to your peers (particularly if you've heard that, as a minority student, you *don't* stack up). You may wonder how you'll handle the competition when you're faced with it head on. Competition can be very helpful and healthy. So rather than just sitting and wondering (or worrying!), you can prepare yourself to manage competition during medical school to your best advantage.

> **Competition:** a contest between rivals.

Your Style

Styles of competition are usually formed by our past experiences, values, and beliefs. We all have experience with it. If your experience has been fun, with rewarding outcomes, you may look forward to competition. If you've had more negative experiences, such as shame or humiliation in the midst of competition, you may be more inclined to withdraw. In addition to our experiences, we have views about competition formed by our cultures, our families, and our personalities. For example, which concept have you grown up believing the most: "It's not nice to compete" or "Willingness to compete is part of playing the game." "If you can't compete you can't play. And if you can't play, you can't stay" (J. Webb, personal communication, March 1999)?

Depending on your usual style of competition, you will probably have a number of different reactions once thrown into the medical school fray. "I can handle anything you throw at me. Don't hold back. Bring it on." "I'm energized by the whole process." "I feel stupid because everyone else is doing so much better than I am in physiology." "I feel guilty about making someone else look bad in lab."

Of course, no one feels one way all the time, but if your reaction is most frequently like the latter two statements, you may find yourself less able to give your all. Your thoughts are tied up in managing uncomfortable feelings rather than focused on the task at hand. So how do you move to a more effective style?

Your Style—Effectively

Your *first step* in finding an effective style is to *identify your rival(s)*. Are they your *individual classmates*—those who brag about how well they are doing so they can intimidate their peers? They may say casually, "You studied *how* long??? I finished that chapter in an hour and went out to a movie." (In reality, they studied all night just like you did. They are just trying to demoralize you). There also may be those who engage you in competition without your consent. They steal a set of histology slides so that the rest of the group cannot study. Is your rival "*the mean*"—the average grade in the class on an exam? Many students feel they've done well only if they've done better than the mean. This translates, "better than the average student." Of course, there is no such student, because the "average" is a number. Even if there was an average student, remember that the average in medical school is pretty darn smart. Are your competitors *stereotypes?* (e.g., that minorities can't handle medical school). Stereotypes are myths and should be treated as such (see Chapter 5). Is it *time*? "I must get all the work done in a certain number of hours."

Determining your competitor is crucial, because your true rival sets the standard for your performance. In track, you win if you run faster than your opponent. If you are trying to beat the other runners, you only run faster than *their* best. You may never run as fast as *you* can (Bernard, 1960). On the other hand, suppose you look at your own test score and see a number of careless errors on the multiple-choice questions. You decide that you will learn to answer questions more judiciously. Or you see that you really blew one entire section. You vow to try to hit all the most important areas next time. In other words, you are competing with your own past performance. *You are your own rival.* You can always reach for your greatest potential; you are in control— not someone/something else.

Second, map out a strategy. If other potential rivals are not the primary focus, you can keep your eyes on the real goal: finding ways to maximize your progress in learning medicine. This will enhance your overall academic work rather than your just blindly shooting for a higher test score. Like it or not, many grades in medical school are subject to the professor's choice of questions, to the performance of other students, and to how well you feel that day. Strategies to improve your test taking or study skills will last long after the exam is over. Hopefully, your scores will improve too, but if they don't, you still profit for future exams.

Summary

Competition is a reality in medical school. Choosing yourself as a rival gives you your best odds of winning.

Maintaining Motivation

One of the most common challenges in the basic science years is that of maintaining motivation. Many students start out "gung ho," fueled by excitement or anxiety. However, maintaining an intense focus over a long period of time is difficult. You can depend on there being a time when you will no longer feel like studying, going to class, or even being in medical school. You will feel like Joe (Webb & Núñez, 1995-1998):

> Joe is bored. He just started the first semester of his second year, and he can't seem to get into it. He did OK during the first year—able to study, interested, and enjoying most of the subjects. He worked on his car, played his horn, and did nothing over the summer; he thought he was ready to start second year. Joe expected Path and ICM to be interesting, but he is sick of going to class already. With exams two weeks away, he still can't get into his work. He wonders how he will ever make it through at this rate.

Almost every human being gets a cold at some time in his or her life. Almost every, if not every, medical student feels unmotivated at some point (or points) during medical school. Why does it happen?

How Motivation Works

The word *motivate* comes from the Latin word *moveo,* to move. Like a child on a swing set, the first push will propel you forward. Your motivation (initial excitement, other's pride, a book) can get you energized for the short term. However, If the child doesn't keep pumping with her own legs, pretty soon the swing will slow to a stop. Or if someone grabs the ropes and slows the swing down, she'll lose her momentum. Movement over the long term has to come from within (Lee, 1998; Lombardi & Baucom, 1997). No one can provide you with motivation for the long term. Motivation is maintained only when you believe in what you are doing and when what you are doing is in line with your goals (Lee, 1998; Lombardi & Baucom, 1997), when you are energized, and when you have hope of success.

There are many reasons why your internal motivation to learn in any setting can be depleted (Wlodkowski & Jaynes, 1991). Your own views of studying and learning affect your motivation. Believing that someone outside you is responsible for your learning, seeing your setbacks as failure (rather than as information to help you learn), fearing the success of your efforts, and being unable to organize your learning, all are elements that can lessen your motivation. Furthermore, motivation draws on a limited supply of energy. That is, motivation to *learn* competes with motivation to socialize, motivation to handle the necessities of life, and motivation to relax. In medical school, you may expend much energy studying with sometimes unsatisfying results. Maybe you aren't getting the A (or B or C) you expected. Or you aren't learning as much as you thought, or the studying seems endless. No wonder you soon find your energy to study depleted.

There are other reasons that motivation wanes. Motivation (Wlodkowski & Jaynes, 1991) is also influenced by cultural values, family values, and teachers. If your family believes education to be a ticket to success, they will likely help motivate you to succeed academically. If they find the opposite, that education was not open to them, they may subtly or directly hinder you (see Chapter 7). There is also pressure imposed by the grading system. If teachers discourage you or show lack of faith in your potential, they may be like those pulling on the ropes of your swing, slowing you down. Because lack of motivation is such a universal phenomenon, you can quit hating yourself for feeling it. You may be tempted to lay the guilt on thick: "People sacrificed so much, and look at me—I'm not even trying." Or "I'm just wasting money." But guilt trips take you nowhere. You may even hear people make subtle references about minorities being lazy. Remember that self-reproach is just one more way to divert your attention from studying. Your energy would be far better spent managing the problem.

Managing Your Motivation

OK, you appreciate and accept your humanness and the inevitability of your attacks of "I just don't feel like studying today." So how can you prepare yourself to deal with them (Webb & Núñez, 1995-1998)?

Preparing for the Lack of Motivation

Your preparation should start with some self-reflection (Webb & Núñez, 1995-1998). The *first question* to ask yourself is "why am I here in medical school?" Beyond the classic interview answer ("to help people,"), why did you come? *Honestly* list for yourself all the reasons—even the ones that are purely utilitarian: interest in biology, desire to make up for illness/death experienced by you or a loved one, the prestige, the money, the lack of any better ideas for a career choice, pressure from others, spiritual calling, and so on. Write everything down.

When you have been brutally honest, ask yourself the *second question:* "What would make me decide to leave?" Resist the temptation to answer "nothing could make me quit." It is not a sign of lack of commitment; you will not "jinx" yourself if you can identify some specific possibilities. Instead, you will likely learn crucial information. After you've done this work, ask the *third question:* "What usually (in life outside of medical school) makes me want to quit?" A task that's too hard? Too easy? A relationship being threatened? Think of the reasons listed above that make motivation wane.

And then the *fourth question:* "What usually makes me want to keep going?" Is it the carrot (promise of a sundae after studying) or the stick (promise of a failure if I don't).

These four questions are windows into what it is that keeps you motivated. They can help you understand why you're not motivated now. And they can provide clues about how to get out of the rut.

What Do I Do?

If you are already in the midst of a work slow down, you must take some *immediate* steps because you just don't have time to stop the train in medical school. Your approach will depend on whether you are unmotivated at the 11th hour or if you have a little time to think (Webb & Núñez, 1995-1998).

When There Is Still a Little Time to Think. If you have some time (e.g., two weeks before exams), you may be able to take a moment to reflect. And if you do, ask yourself what's stopping you from working. Are you *sick of the studying itself* (too much continuous intensity) or is there more to it? You may get some hints from your answers to Questions 2 and 3 above.

"I hate this stuff." Remember that wanting to be a doctor should not be confused with liking the thing you're studying at the moment. It may be that you and this subject were just not meant to be related by more than necessity. And as long as you learn what's required, that's enough. *Fear of doing poorly* can be a motivator, but it can also paralyze you. Or it may cause you to just give up. In either case, the fear is now in control, and that's the thing to address. On the other hand, recognition that "no matter what, I'll pass" or "I always seem to get the same grade no matter how much I study" can also demotivate. Another demotivator is *"medical school overdose."* Thinking about medicine all the time with little other input can cause anyone distress. Sometimes, the

demotivator is a "who." *Other unmotivated medical student friends* or friends who aren't in school at all sometimes urge you to other pursuits. Or *people who are* just the opposite—*"too intense"* about school. These students can be exhausting, and too much contact with them may cause you to lose what little energy you have. Especially watch out for a particular breed: those *people who think you can't make it.* You may be ready for those people who are not your friends. But occasionally, there also may be old classmates from home who are jealous of your success or other medical students competing against you or professors who wonder if *any* minority student can make it. Occasionally, a spouse or a parent may have little faith in you. Because people often communicate this opinion nonverbally, you may not be immediately aware of the impact of their presence.

Any of these feelings or people can decrease your motivation. If you have time to figure out who or what is the culprit, you can go right to the source. Here is where your answers to Questions 1 and 4 above are helpful. One student volunteered two hours a week at the Salvation Army Clinic to stay in touch with patients. Alter your approach to a subject you hate; just get the facts down—don't waste time trying to love it. Compartmentalize your fears: "I have one job now: learning the material. If I worry about the grade, I'll stop doing my job." If the fear is deeply rooted, consider talking it through with a trusted counselor or psychiatrist. And simply put, stay away from discouraging people.

At the 11th Hour. If, on the other hand, this is the 11th hour, you will need a different approach. The night before the exam, there's obviously no time for soul searching. Now you need to act. The key is *change.* Change your location. Leave the library or your apartment and go somewhere else to study. Change your company. Find someone to study with or along side of you. (Tell yourself, "I'm not in this by myself.") Cut loose those who bring you down. Or change your method of study. Start from the end of the lecture notes. Make note cards. Schedule more frequent breaks (every 15 minutes if necessary). And up the ante; increase the number of rewards for your accomplishments (two pieces of chocolate every time you finish a chapter). Do anything. Just change, because the status quo isn't working.

Summary

The more you understand why you are unmotivated, the more accurately you can identify a solution. Don't wait to implement your options.

The USMLE:
Meeting "Standardized" Challenges

The USMLE (U.S. Medical Licensure Examination) is the universal tool of medical education to assess the knowledge and skills attainment levels of graduates and practitioners. Accrediting organizations also use it as an external measure of the success of medical schools' training programs. Do not view it as punitive or as a "negative control" designed to deny you and other graduates entrée into medicine.

The various steps (achievement levels) in medical education training are tested using Steps 1, 2, and 3 of the USMLE. USMLE Step 1 tests your grasp of the basic science years. Most medical schools require that you pass it prior to entering the junior (third) year. In addition, most schools require passage of USMLE Step 2 (which gauges your clinical knowledge) to be awarded the Doctor of Medicine (M.D.) degree. Finally, practical application of your skills is tested by USMLE Step 3 during the first year of residency.

When Do You Begin Reviews for the USMLE?

So when do you begin preparation for passing USMLE Steps 1 and 2? Establish your approach from Day 1—integrating the material you learn. Integrate the biochemistry of glucose production with the physiology of muscle movement. You will be building on your medical knowledge and taking comprehensive exams for the remainder of your career. So make this practice of integration a professional *lifestyle* change. Some form of formal review should start no later than the end of the first academic year. During the summer following the first year, you should assess your knowledge level. This is not difficult to do if you take advantage of the learning resources available. For example, many basic science departments opt to administer the NBME (National Board of Medical Examiners) shelf exams. These exams follow the USMLE format but include questions retired from the USMLE question bank. Most medical schools have learning resource centers that offer computer-based self-assessment modules in all the basic science courses. You should always retain copies of departmental course examinations and answer keys. Using these tools, you should be able to ascertain the relative level of your ability to pass a comprehensive examination.

During the second year, you should be integrating your knowledge from first year with that of second year and begin to see relationships between biochemistry and pharmacology, microbiology and pathology, and so on. During the winter holidays of the second year, take time to develop a comprehensive study schedule. It should emphasize topics in your weakest areas. During the second semester of the second year, you should spend a few hours every week reviewing these topics.

The USMLE administers Steps 1, 2, and 3 on computer. So get as comfortable as possible with a computer before you take the exam. Consider: If you had to stop and think about how to use a pencil during an exam, your test taking would slow down considerably. Obviously, owning your own computer and/or having access to e-mail and the Internet will broaden your access to learning resources and instructional faculty.

Most schools expect you to sit for the USMLE Step 2 in the fall of your senior year, and they use your results to determine whether you graduate. You'll have less time to study for this one, so it is critical that you maintain an active recall of knowledge. Your departmental or NBME shelf exams after each rotation will give you a good idea of your level of factual knowledge. Ask fourth-year students with records like yours to share specific approaches they used to prepare for it.

Examination Format and Approaches to Study

The format of questions on the USMLE is a very public piece of information (of course, the questions on the examination are not). You'll want to get good at demonstrating your knowledge in this format. So during *each study period,* use review books and practice exams to *do questions.* Ask upper years in your institution how much you can rely on lecture notes and departmental exams to prepare for the USMLE. Word of caution: The self-study approach is economical and effective *if* you have the personal discipline and time management skills to make it work for you. Alternatively, you will be inundated with announcements about medical school-based or commercial prep courses available. Some even guarantee passage of the exam using their approach. Some schools will offer financial assistance to help you prepare for the examination. Weigh all your options carefully and make your own choice about the approach. You should be willing to live with the decision you make regardless of the outcome of your performance on the examination.

Preparing Your Mind-Set

Anticipation of the USMLE is one of the primary factors that makes second year so stressful. Because of the widely disseminated belief that "minority students can't do well on standardized tests" (see Chapter 5) and depending on your own track record on this type of exam, you may be particularly apprehensive, if not downright terrified about it. Yes, this exam is important. So preparing your mind to deal with the exam is even more important.

Hindrances to Your Studying

Consider the following concerns medical students have had in the midst of studying for the USMLE:

I don't know what areas they emphasize in physiology.

I can't figure out what they meant by that sample question.

I wish I knew what they wanted on this one.

If you've ever made these comments or ones like them, ask yourself a question. Who are "they?" If they are "Board people," then take a minute to visualize the Board people. Who do you see? For many minorities, it is an image similar to the one this student describes:

The Board is probably a group of gray-haired, White men (maybe some women). At best, they are designing an exam with only the majority student in mind. At worst, the group is racist, wanting all minority students to fail, and writing the test questions for *that* purpose.

Maybe this particular image does not hit home, but consider carefully your *mental picture of the people making up the test.* You can see how much the above picture would put you in a "one down" position for the boards. You will be walking into the exam, not to show off your knowledge, but to fight against stereotypes. And if the whole system of the boards is designed that way, your chances of winning may seem hopeless.

Another hindrance to your attitude is the rumor mill.

Black male second-year medical student to Black faculty member: "Is it true that, over half the minorities across the country who took the USMLE last year failed it?"

Rumors of who passes in your state, your school, your race/gender/ ethnicity will abound. Remember that those statistics are more useful for institutions planning curriculum and academic support services than for you predicting your own performance. Whether the statistics point to your success or your failure does not change the bottom line: You need to study. And statistics for everyone else won't change one bit how much *you* need to study.

Another huge hindrance to studying is your *state of exhaustion* in the second semester of second year. This is typically a time of being sick of studying, of classmates, of your school, of everything related to medicine. If you aren't turned on by the limited patient contact, you may feel extremely discouraged about what's ahead. So to be asked to add USMLE preparation on top of all this could feel like needles under your fingernails. It's extremely important to have a schedule—and to stick with it even when you don't feel like it.

A further hindrance is *fear of failing.* The consequences of failing are retaking the exam and postponing the continuance of the clinical years. Explore your worst fears. What would it mean to you to postpone your rotations? Is it the money? The responses of family/friends/professors/classmates? The time? Do some reality testing and anticipatory problem solving. You may want to use a counselor to put your apprehension in perspective. If you do not understand the reality of your concerns, your fear may take over.

Less frequently, you may be hindered because you *underestimate the importance of the exam* or the need to study early. You have nothing to lose by studying. And everything to lose if you don't. As one student lamented after failing Step 2 of the boards,

> I just didn't study enough. I had done well on USMLE Step 1 and done fine on my rotations. I believed my classmates when they told me the guidelines for preparation time. Step 1—study 4 weeks. Step 2—study two weeks. Step 3—Number 2 pencil. Now I have to take it again.

Adjusting to Your Mind-Set

To make it through this study period, start with an attitude change—not necessarily using positive thinking (I'm going to pass) or negative thinking (I'm going to fail) but using reality thinking: "This exam will measure my ability to answer basic science questions from a question bank on a given day. It is not a measure of my potential to be a good doctor" (see Chapter 5).

"Studying is my opportunity to synthesize the information I've learned so far. The exam is my opportunity to display my knowledge in a particular format."

Test Time: What Do You Do When You Get to the Test?

You should enter the testing center with a strategy in mind for taking the examination, much like a businessperson entering a room to run a meeting. For example, based on what worked for you on practice exams, you'll read questions twice, underline key words, mark "b" if you don't know the answer, and so on. For each question, you should try to explain to yourself why you chose the answer you did, referring (in your mind) to the source materials from which your answer was derived (e.g., notes, text). As you move through the exam, pace yourself. When you come to a question (or a series of questions!) that you can't answer, take a mental break and a breath, and move on. This is not the time for predictions (I know I'm going to fail) but for working on questions.

If You Receive a Failing Grade

If you do not pass the USMLE, you will experience myriad feelings. Some students are shocked; others are embarrassed and worried about what others will think of them. Some are angry at the examiners. Some feel shame, guilt at letting people down, or anxiety about getting into a residency. As a result of these feelings, all too commonly, students will hide. It is imperative that after you have given yourself a few days to process the news, you tell someone (who'll offer you support) that you didn't pass the exam. Next, contact medical education, minority affairs, or the right school office to find out your next steps. Then begin to tell others who care about you. It is not that your performance is necessarily their business. But keeping this information a secret from key administrators (who are bound to find out anyway) will create and magnify feelings of shame. It also prevents you from getting support or from planning your strategy for next time.

Summary

The USMLE is a challenging but very do-able milestone in your basic science years. Because you will commit so much time and energy to preparing for it, approach it as your opportunity to consolidate your knowledge and recognize areas for improvement.

Conclusion

The basic science years are filled with excitement and challenge. Your diligence and flexibility in managing the material and the culture will play heavily in your performance.

REFERENCES

Becker, H., Geer, B., Hughes, E. C., & Strauss, A. C. (1961). *Boys in white.* New Brunswick, NJ: Transaction Publishers.

Bernard, J. (1960, January). Autonomic and decisive forms of competition. *Sociological Quarterly,* 25-35.

Committee on Education, Group for Advancement of Psychiatry. (1982). *A survival manual for medical students.* New York: Mental Health Materials Center.

Fine, P. (1994). *The wards.* Boston: Little, Brown.

Galanti, G.-A. (1991). *Caring for patients from different cultures.* Philadelphia: University of Pennsylvania Press.

Kaplan, H. I., & Sadock, B. J. (1989). *Comprehensive textbook of psychiatry* (Vol. 2). Baltimore: Williams & Wilkins.

Lee, B. (1998). *The power principle.* New York: Simon & Schuster.

Lombardi, V. Jr., & Baucom, J. (1997). *Baby steps to success.* Lancaster, PA: Starburst.

Myers, M. F. (1998). Words of wisdom. *BC Medical Journal, 40*(11), 496-517.

Shields, P. H. (1994). A survey and analysis of student academic support programs in medical schools. Focus: Underrepresented minority students. *Journal of the National Medical Association, 86,* 373-377.

Stein, H. F. (1990). *American medicine as culture.* Boulder, CO: Westview.

Webb, C., & Núñez, A. (1995-1998). Non-cognitive tools. In A. Núñez & C. Webb (Eds.), *Navigating the medical culture: Medical student course curricular document.* Philadelphia, PA: MCP Hahnemann University. (Available from the authors)

Wlodkowski, R. J., & Jaynes, J. H. (1991). *Eager to learn: Helping children become motivated and love learning.* San Francisco: Jossey-Bass.

3 Life on the Wards

When all the Rules Change

MARGARITA HAUSER GARDINER, MD

By the time you reach the third year of medical school, you have had some contact with patients, if only during the process of learning how to take medical histories and perform physical examinations. The third and fourth years— the clinical years—are, however, fundamentally different from the previous, preclinical years. During the first two years, you are charged with committing to memory factual knowledge about the human body, what it's made of, how it works normally, how it works abnormally, and how chemicals can be used to alter normal and abnormal function. In most schools, this process is primarily a didactic one: lecturers lecture, students read, and examinations are given. In others, learning is more self-directed, with individual students or groups of students charged with the responsibility of discovering what they need to know and then learning the material. During the clinical years, however, learning is driven by experience with patients. Furthermore, although you are expected to learn how to diagnose and treat illness, you are also expected to function as a working member of a team of physicians and students. Rules of learning change; so do rules of dress, behavior, and evaluation.

Students from minority groups underrepresented in medicine frequently do well in this setting. Clinical success depends heavily on problem-solving skills, which most students of color have used to reach this level. Moreover, many patients admitted to hospital teaching services are medically disenfranchised and are more comfortable sharing important information with medical students whom they perceive are also disenfranchised.

To excel during these years, you must know the new rules, including who is involved and what the expectations are. This chapter is designed to (a) describe the categories of people with whom you will interact, (b) define your role, (c) identify some pitfalls that await students of color, and (d) offer some suggestions for navigating rough seas. Problems *will* arise, and the best defenses for students of color are competence and professionalism.

PART I: THE NEW RULES

Clinical Clerkships

During the third year, the course work is divided into clinical rotations, most of which are hospital based, covering the basic medical disciplines: medicine, surgery, neurology, psychiatry, pediatrics, obstetrics, and gynecology. The fourth year consists of required and elective courses, which provide exposure to specialties and subspecialties.

You are graded on factual knowledge, ability to integrate data, problem solving, and teamwork. One of the most difficult things to accept is that your grade is usually based on subjective evaluations from those who are teaching you, as well as—for required courses—performance on written examinations. The determinants vary from school to school, but they usually include knowledge of the subject, verbal and written communication, professionalism, and teamwork.

Because the process *is* somewhat subjective, you may sometimes feel you have been graded unfairly. You may wonder whether a poor or mediocre evaluation is based on racial or cultural factors rather than on your performance. A poor subjective evaluation, unlike a poor score on a standardized examination, may cause an emotional response: You may feel rejected or excluded from a group whose mores you don't understand. In such a system, you must have a clear understanding of what is expected of you at the outset.

When a patient is admitted to a hospital, the patient is assigned to a primary service, according to the type of care required. Most general hospitals have medical and surgical services; many have pediatric, obstetrical, gynecologic, psychiatric, or neurological services. Services may be further classified according to subspecialty, such as orthopedic surgery or cardiology. There may also be critical care or intensive care units. Consultants may provide additional care.

As you move from one service to another or from one level of care to another, you will find that the cultures and the expectations change, sometimes dramatically. You must approach each new assignment with flexibility and an open mind and adapt quickly to the new environment.

Who's Who

When you are assigned to a service, you are part of a team whose members have specific roles and different levels of responsibility. Although there may be variations in the number and relative ranks of the team members, the hierarchy referred to in Chapter 1 is very clearly defined.

Attending Physician. The attending physician (usually referred to as the attending) is the physician who is legally responsible for the patient's care—the ultimate decision-making authority. He or she may teach the residents and students who are caring for the patients on his or her service; if so, the attending will be required to evaluate you. This evaluation contributes to the grade you receive for the course and may be considered by the dean when writing the letter of recommendation, which accompanies your application for residency. The attending may also write independent letters of recommendation.

Teaching Resident. The teaching resident is a physician-in-training who has completed at least one year of postgraduate training. He or she supervises and teaches the first-year residents (interns) and a medical student assigned to the service and participates in grading you.

Intern. The intern, or first-year resident, is a physician in the first year of training following graduation from medical school. The intern evaluates the patient at the time of admission and is then responsible for the day-to-day care of the patient. The intern teaches you the basics of patient care. From your intern, you learn how to write progress notes, enter orders in the chart, perform basic procedures (such as obtaining blood, urine, and sputum samples and inserting intravenous catheters) and write prescriptions for patients at the time of discharge. Depending on the service, the intern also teaches you more specialized procedures, such as dressing changes or suture removal.

Subintern. The subintern is a fourth-year medical student who, with the close supervision of the resident, performs some of the duties of an intern. The subintern has no formal teaching responsibilities but may be a source of information and assistance to you during your third year.

Nursing Personnel. Do not underestimate the importance of nursing personnel as active participants in your education. Nurses are vital members of the patient care team and are sources of valuable information, including drug dosing, wound care, and the locations of supplies and equipment. Nurses can help you avoid embarrassing or potentially dangerous errors. If you treat nurses with respect rather than with disdain or condescension, your life on the ward will be much easier.

Ancillary Personnel. There are many people who interact with hospitalized patients on a daily basis, and you will come into contact with most of them. Laboratory technicians obtain blood samples, respiratory technicians administer breathing treatments, orderlies transport patients, dietary aides transport trays, and so on, although in some hospitals, nurses or care assistants perform some of or all these functions. Most hospitals employ physical, occupational, and speech therapists, who help patients regain lost or impaired function. Social workers assist patients with insurance, transportation home, child care, domestic violence intervention, facilitation of discharge or transfer to other institutions, and other related issues.

Ancillary personnel are integral to the smooth operation of the hospital and to the comfort and well-being of the patients, and they deserve your respect. In some settings, many service workers are members of minority groups. Your shared background may lead to displays of familiarity, which are not appropriate in a professional setting. If, however, you do not respond in the hospital the same way that you would in a casual or recreational setting, you may be thought of as arrogant or as having abandoned your origins. To navigate this potential minefield, maintain an attitude of professionalism *and* cordiality at all times.

Patient. The patient is the most important—and, potentially, the most frightening—person with whom you will have contact. The patient is the reason for the whole system: medical school, hospital, residency. The patient also represents the awesome privilege and responsibility of being a physician.

The Daily Routine

The Medical Record. The "chart" is the repository of information about the patient's hospital course. It is a medical *and* a legal document. Any event that is recorded in the medical record is presumed to have actually happened, and any event that is not recorded is presumed *not* to have happened. This is an important concept and may be a difficult one for students accustomed to oral-based cultural systems (see Chapter 1). The section on oral and written communication will expand on this.

Access to the medical record is officially restricted to those who have a legitimate interest and involvement in the care of the patient. Practically speaking, however, anyone who has access to the working areas of a hospital unit has physical access to the patient's chart. Entries into the medical record are made by those personnel who have substantive interactions with the patient. The entries made by medical students are, for the most part, "progress notes," narrative records of ongoing events. Your notes are very important. *They are a primary representation of your skill as a clinician and may be the only basis for the impression some physicians form of you.* The student note is usually the most detailed and most legible one in the chart and is frequently consulted by others who want a factual account of the patient's progress. Don't let anyone tell you that no one ever looks at the medical student note; always assume that anything you write in the chart will be reviewed and critiqued by *everyone* who is involved in the patient's care!

The Workday: Structured Time

Work Rounds. Residents and students discuss each patient's status and form a daily plan of action. This is your opportunity to learn the nuts and bolts of managing patients, so be *on time* and *prepared.*

Attending Rounds. If the attending makes formal teaching rounds, this is the time when you present patients to him or her. The presentation is a structured verbal report of the patient's status and the tentative plans for patient care activities. The attending quizzes the team and provides instruction.

Procedures. On surgical services, you are expected to be present in the operating room to assist with surgical procedures, including obstetrical deliveries.

Teaching Conferences. You are generally expected to attend all conferences held for the service to which you are assigned.

Outpatient Activities. You may be expected to accompany residents to the outpatient clinics to see patients or to accompany attending physicians during office hours.

The Workday: Unstructured Time

Unstructured time includes your day-to-day activities, self-directed learning, and time spent "on-call" (time spent in the hospital, usually overnight, during which you admit patients and see to the needs of patients whose teams have left the hospital). Some activities are performed with the other members of the team; others are performed independently. These activities include, but are not limited to, the following:

- Seeing previously assigned patients and writing progress notes
- Evaluating newly admitted patients and recording each new patient's medical history and physical examination findings
- Retrieving data
- Performing procedures
- Reading

It is sometimes difficult to manage unstructured time well. You will be tempted to take advantage of "down time," when you are not actively involved in patient care duties, to relax and socialize with other students or nursing personnel rather than to study or review material. Remember that as a person of color, you are highly visible; even if you are part of a group of students who appear to be "goofing off," you may well be the only individual clearly identified by your resident or attending.

Student Responsibilities

Assigned Patients. When a newly admitted patient is assigned to you, you will take a detailed medical history (H) and perform a complete physical examination (P). This may be accomplished independently or in the presence of the intern. The written H&P is, ideally, reviewed and cosigned by the attending physician, who, again ideally, may critique it. If a patient is transferred to your team and assigned to you, you are expected to review the chart, examine the patient, and write a progress note summarizing the events preceding the transfer and recording your physical findings.

You are expected to visit each assigned patient at the beginning of the day, obtain a brief interval history, and perform a limited physical examination; then you gather information that has accumulated since the previous day's rounds. *You* are the designated source of information about *your* patients for the rest of the team. If you repeatedly fail to have the needed information during rounds, you are viewed as lazy and disinterested as well as an embarrassment to the rest of the team.

You write the daily progress note in a prescribed format for each assigned patient. You also write orders in the chart; initially, this is done under close supervision. An intern or resident must cosign your progress notes and orders. (Don't worry, no one will respond to your orders unless they are cosigned by a physician!)

When your patient is discharged, you complete the necessary paperwork, including any needed prescriptions (which will be cosigned). You may also be expected to make arrangements, even appointments, for outpatient follow-up.

Teamwork. As a member of the team, you may be asked to assist the intern or resident in performing tasks which are not directly related to your assigned patients. There is a certain amount of "scut" (*s*ub *c*ortical *u*tilization of *t*ime) work that must be done on a daily basis, and well-operated teams get this work done on a cooperative basis. There is learning value in almost everything you do; some residents, however, will take unfair advantage of you when assigning such tasks. Unless you are being so overburdened by scut work that you have no time for reading, it probably doesn't pay to complain.

If the amount of work assigned to you seems unreasonable, you should probably check with the clerkship director before bringing it up with the team. If you *do* decide to complain, ask to speak to your resident privately. Try to voice your concerns in terms of your overall learning experience, as in, "I'm really learning a lot about dressing changes, but I need a little more time to read about my patients." If you start off by complaining about the amount of work you are doing, you will appear to be lazy and uncooperative. From the point of view of the resident and intern, the best medical student is one who unburdens the rest of the team by actively participating in patient care.

Self-Directed Learning. During the clinical years, you are responsible for learning as much as possible about the diagnosis and management of the diseases presented by the patients on the team. You *must* keep up with your reading. For the most part, no one will assign reading to you. It is up to you to read early and often about as many of the diagnoses discussed by your team as possible. Don't confine your reading to your own patients; pay attention to the diseases managed by the rest of the team. You may be expected to demonstrate what has been learned by making informal oral presentations about a particular disease during rounds or by making a more formal presentation at a conference. Learn to conform to the norms of medical culture: Your presentations must be succinct and informative, precise and pertinent. This is not oratory; this is scientific communication.

Expectations. It is a frightening and unsettling experience to enter the clinical years without having a clear understanding of what is expected of you by all the parties involved. Sometimes, it is *knowing* what is expected that is frightening!

Patients who are not familiar with the routines of a teaching hospital may not understand your role. Some patients assume that you are a physician; others express resentment that they are being cared for, even in part, by students and consider themselves to be unwilling experimental subjects. You should make it clear that you are *not* a physician but, rather, a student doctor working with a team of doctors.

Some residents and interns take their teaching responsibilities very seriously and enjoy the opportunity to share their skills with students. Others view students as necessary appendages who exist primarily to do work that the intern doesn't want to do. Still others don't want to be bothered at all. They all, however, expect you to see assigned patients, write notes, and perform assigned tasks. They also expect you not to embarrass them on rounds by being late, inarticulate, or unprepared.

The attending physician expects you to be present and on time, to know current details about assigned patients, to have basic knowledge about the disease under discussion, and to make fluent, coherent, well-organized oral presentations.

The importance of being on time and prepared for rounds cannot be overemphasized. If rounds begin at 7:00 a.m., you *must* arrive early enough to see your patients, make note of any events that have occurred since the previous day's rounds, record available data, and prepare yourself to present promptly at 7:00 a.m. Even if a resident, an intern, another student, or even the attending physician is usually late, *you* must be on time and prepared. It is a fact of life for persons of color that we are conspicuous in such settings; your tardiness or lack of preparation will stand out!

Absences are sometimes unavoidable, but you should make every effort to schedule car repairs, dental visits, or parent-teacher conferences at times that do not conflict with rounds. The attending physician has probably rearranged his or her office or operating schedule to make time for rounds and will likely notice and resent your absence. The resident may view absences as evidence of disinterest or lack of motivation, and this will be reflected in your course evaluation.

PART II: WHEN THINGS GO WRONG

Some of the problem situations that will arise may occur for all students, others primarily for students of color. Whatever the situation, it is important to recognize the problem and take steps to resolve it promptly; otherwise, you will be distracted from the business of caring for your patients and learning medicine.

Stumbling Blocks

The following examples are drawn from the author's experiences during medical school and residency and from the experiences of students mentored by the author.

Patient Relations

A fourth-year student of color taking a senior elective was asked to see a patient in consultation. He went into the patient's room, introduced himself, and stated the reason for his visit. The patient, a 50-year-old White woman, looked at him, said, "I'd rather have someone else," and turned her face to the wall.

It is rare that a patient will overtly refuse to be assigned to a student of a different race, but it does happen. The rejection may be subtle. The patient may refuse to make eye contact or answer questions, or resist examination, only to be fully interactive and cooperative with a resident who is *not* a person of color. Nothing overt has happened here, but you are left feeling inadequate and, possibly, appearing incompetent. Moreover, it is difficult to extricate yourself from such a situation without seeming to be petty, as in "Mrs. A just won't talk to me the way she talks to you," or even worse, lazy, "Maybe you should assign Mrs. A to someone else." The best approach here is to continue to do what you are supposed to do: Ask the questions; perform the examination, if possible; track down the data; then present the information. If necessary, you may need to document, *objectively,* in the chart that the patient would not permit an examination. Don't editorialize or make subjective comments here; a factual statement, such as "patient refused physical examination" is appropriate and sufficient.

On the other hand, patients who identify strongly with you may communicate with you to the exclusion of other members of the team. In most cases, the team will respect the relationship between you and the patient, but an insecure house officer may resent it. Sometimes, the other team members may assume that because you share the patient's cultural background, you may be able to communicate more effectively with the patient. You may be comfortable accepting this role; if not, you may want to state, again objectively, that the patient is no more willing to talk to you than he or she is to anyone else on the team. Occasionally, a patient may inappropriately express admiration, sexual attraction, or a desire to pursue a relationship with you outside the medical setting. This is not necessarily "harassment," but it can be uncomfortable or even offensive. The most effective response here is to state clearly and matter-of-factly that a personal relationship is inappropriate, return the conversation to the matter at hand, complete the task in process, and leave the scene. You may wish to ask a third person, perhaps a nurse, aide, or another student, to be present during future encounters with the patient.

Exclusionary Tactics

A-third-year medical student was the only minority member of a group of six students assigned to the general surgery service at a community hospital. By the end of the second week of the six-week rotation, it was clear that the other members of the group were spending much more time in the operating room than she was and that she was spending much more time doing dressing changes than they were. She was very concerned about this, because she was missing an important part of the rotation and was at risk of receiving a poor evaluation from the attending physician. She spoke to her intern, who shrugged and indicated that it was simply the luck of the draw that resulted in her not being assigned patients who required surgery. She then approached the chief resident and asked him to review the procedure logs of all the students, explaining that she felt she was not doing her share of OR time. In this case, the resident was receptive and agreed that more attention should be paid to distributing cases evenly.

This is a difficult sort of situation in which the racial exclusion is subtle and difficult to define or to prove. Moreover, complaints of being excluded are likely to result in your being labeled a "whiner" or someone who doesn't like to perform menial tasks. The student's approach here, basing her case on facts (the number of procedures observed by each student) was effective. Sometimes, however, this doesn't work, particularly if the person to whom the appeal is made is actively participating in the exclusion. You may need to discuss the situation with the clerkship director, broaching the subject in terms of the breadth of the learning situation rather than in terms of being locked out of the group. You might open the discussion by saying, "I don't think I'm seeing as many types of surgical procedures as I need to," or "How can I get more OR time?," then follow with your assessment of the situation.

The Inquisition

The third-year students are participating in the professor's rounds. A White male student stands and presents the case to the professor, who is the chairman of the department, then is allowed to take his seat. A Puerto Rican woman, visibly nervous, is called to the front to interpret a chest X-ray. She begins to speak, barely audibly, and is interrupted by the professor. "Well," he says acidly, "can you tell us what part of the body this is?" "Chest, Doctor," she replies. "Can you name an organ found in the chest?" "Lung, Doctor." "Very good! Now, do you think you can show us a lung?" The student bolts from the room in tears.

One of the more unpleasant aspects of life on the wards is the frequent use of the Socratic teaching method. The teacher and student engage in a question-and-answer session, with the questions becoming more difficult and complex until the student's knowledge of the subject has been exhausted and he or she can no longer answer correctly. Some students are comfortable with this method; most are not. Everyone gets exposed to it, however, and few are unscathed by it, regardless of racial or cultural background.

In this instance, the Puerto Rican student felt that she was being unfairly attacked by the professor, who had not quizzed the White male student at all. More than likely, the professor's motives were not racial; many students have been reduced to tears by aggressive questioning. Those who are uncomfortable with or unaccustomed to speaking before groups are most vulnerable. It is difficult *not* to react as if to a personal attack, but the reality is that nearly everyone is treated in this manner. Some students have more difficulty than others processing the experience in this context and may need to seek help in coping from an academic counselor.

The Bad Grade

An African American student has completed her pediatric rotation at an affiliated hospital in a suburban community. She had chosen the site after consulting with the course director. Most of the patients assigned to her were the children of migrant workers employed at nearby mushroom farms. She worked hard at establishing rapport with the patients and their families and spent extra time in the office of one of the attending pediatricians. She thought she was doing a good job, and she scored well on the written examination. Several months later, when she went to her adviser to review her course evaluation, she was surprised to find that, although her grade was good and most of the comments were positive, she was referred to as "manipulative" and "not a team player." She was very upset, because she was afraid that the tone of the evaluation would influence her dean's letter of recommendation. She had planned to ask for a letter of recommendation from the attending and was now reluctant to do so.

It is probable that the student did not seek periodic feedback from the resident and attending physician. More than likely, the negative comments came from the resident, who may have been resentful of the student's close relationships with the patients and with the attending physician. The student sought the advice of her adviser, who knew her well. The adviser offered to contact the attending, but the student felt comfortable doing this herself. The attending assured her that he had graded her positively and that he would be pleased to write a letter of recommendation for her. He then spoke to the clerkship director, who persuaded the resident to amend the negative comments.

Your course evaluation is critical; it is very important to solicit feedback early in the rotation and, if necessary, involve the attending physician in remediating any perceived weaknesses. Where many students go wrong is in not seeking advice and assistance. By getting acquainted with her adviser and by establishing contact with the course director, the student in this situation had, in effect, set up her appeals court before she knew she would need it.

Social Commentary

Scene 1 A medical student of mixed race is the only student of color currently taking her third-year gynecology rotation. The last three patients were very young African American women who were treated for sexually transmitted diseases. As the students are leaving the clinic area, one comments that the Tuskegee Experiment had been terminated too soon.

Scene 2 Two students, one African American, one White, are comparing notes about their experiences in two different hospitals. The first hospital was a Veteran's hospital located in a large urban area, with a largely African American and Puerto Rican patient base. The second was a suburban community hospital with a predominantly White, privately insured population. The White student says, "I'm so glad to be here at (the suburban hospital); I've finally met patients I can relate to. What about you?"

Scene 3 A fourth-year student is discussing with a resident a patient on the hematology consultation service. The patient has sickle cell anemia and is having a painful crisis; the service has been consulted to help control the patient's pain. The resident remarks, "Well, you know these sicklers are all drug seekers. It doesn't really matter what you give them as long as it's a narcotic."

Life as a clinician exposes you to all sorts of thoughtless, and even cruel, comments. In many ways, the group ethos of physicians transcends cultural identity, and colleagues may begin to see one another as primarily members of the group "physicians" and secondarily as members of other ethnic or cultural groups. With this group identity comes a lack of appreciation for distinctions within the group, and colleagues may be genuinely surprised that other physicians—and medical students—are hurt and offended by their remarks. The response depends on what the offended party is trying to accomplish.

Most of us have had quite enough of serving as subjects of socialization for our unenlightened colleagues and lack the stomach and the will to take the opportunity to educate the thoughtless one. Sometimes, as in the first example, the remark is so hurtful that a reasonable response is impossible on the spot; sometimes, as in the second, it is so foolish that ignoring it—and the person who offered it—is the most reasonable course. Sometimes, however, the speaker reveals a level of misinformation, which can cause harm to others, and must be corrected. In a situation like the third one, for example, you might offer factual information, such as, "I've read that chronic pain patients often need high doses of narcotics because narcotics induce tolerance." Another approach is to diplomatically place the speaker in the position of defending his or her position, as in, "Can you suggest an article that supports that statement?" Whatever the response, it is most effective if made objectively and with dignity.

Effective Defensive Strategies

Choose Your Battles Wisely

No one has the time, energy, or credibility to fight for every principle. Some issues are substantive and materially affect your learning, progress, or ability to care for patients. Such issues should and must be addressed promptly. Other issues, while they may be uncomfortable or even hurtful, are less important overall, and must be set aside. The best defense against racially and culturally based attacks, whether subtle or overt, is to be thorough, prepared, and professional.

Identify the Chain of Command

Many students feel that the resident is the most powerful person on the team; you may fear that speaking up for yourself or appealing to a higher authority will jeopardize your grade and/or course evaluation. Although it is true that a resentful resident can make your life miserable, residents don't write letters of recommendation for seniors who are applying to residency; attending physicians, advisers, and deans do. If there is a serious problem with the resident on the service, you can and should approach the attending physician. If you feel that the attending is unapproachable, unsympathetic, or part of the problem, you should appeal to the course director and further, if necessary, to the dean. Again, choose wisely; if you run into the same type of problem on every clinical rotation, you won't have much credibility the third or fourth time you show up in the dean's office.

Use the Support System

Medical students are notorious for underusing their clinical advisers. Most advisers never see the students assigned to them until the senior year is well underway. If an adviser is assigned to you, make a get-acquainted appointment with him or her as soon as the assignment is made, and make frequent contact to let the adviser know how you are faring. If your adviser knows you well, he or she will be more likely to intervene if necessary and will be a more effective advocate. If the adviser is someone with whom you cannot establish rapport and trust, it is better to discover this early on, so that you can find a substitute. Ask the upperclassmen what their experiences have been with advisers; a faculty member who has a reputation for being accessible and helpful to other underrepresented minority students may be willing to counsel you, if not accept you as an official "advisee." A resident with whom you have good rapport may also be able to steer you in the direction of a helpful faculty member.

Find a Mentor

Some students find it useful to identify a faculty member or a physician affiliated with the teaching hospital who will serve as a clinical mentor and a sounding board. This person may or may not be the officially designated adviser. Many community-based physicians and affiliated staff members are quite willing to serve as mentors but may assume that their guidance is not wanted or needed unless requested. Strategies for locating a mentor are discussed in Chapter 7.

Put Your Best Foot Forward

Most of the people involved in your medical education want you to do well. Unfortunately, there are those who expect members of minority groups to fail, and some of *those* will be watching very carefully for telltale signs that you don't belong in medical school. No, it *isn't* fair, but it *is* real and has to be dealt with. In most teaching hospitals, physicians and medical students of color are highly visible, and mistakes take on added significance. Besides, you are embarking on a career in which the well-being of others may depend on your competence; it *is important to strive for excellence whether or not anyone is watching you.*

Dress neatly and appropriately for a workplace, with an appearance that inspires trust and confidence among patients and colleagues; hospital "scrubs" and white coats should be clean and well maintained. Styles of dress and ornamented body parts that may be important media of cultural expression for you may cause patients not to take you seriously as a health care professional.

Be on time for rounds and be prepared with relevant data and other information. Again, the importance of being on time for rounds cannot be overemphasized.

Avoid making excuses; mistakes and omissions should be acknowledged promptly and readily, and data should never be "fudged" or guessed at.

Make oral presentations fluently and concisely, stay with the H&P format taught during the second year, and avoid omissions and backtracking; language should be precise, without idiomatic speech, slang, oratorical style, or dramatization.

Strike Preemptively

Students who receive less than desirable evaluations in clinical courses frequently express surprise and dismay, claiming that they had no idea they were performing poorly. The resident and the attending should point out deficiencies as they are noted, but this does not always happen. Sometimes the feedback is given, but the delivery is subtle. If, for example, the attending or resident interrupts your presentation for clarification or correction, you should make note of it and edit the next presentation accordingly. No later than midway through the rotation you should ask for feedback. The request should be specific, as in "How are my presentations?" or "Is there an area of the physical examination I should be working on?" rather than a general "How am I doing?" When you solicit criticism, however, be prepared to accept and use it; don't react as if you have been personally attacked.

Balance Your Life

Bad things happen all the time. Students oversleep and show up late and unprepared for rounds. Patients die. Attending physicians subject well-meaning students to intense public scrutiny. Snubs and insults and petty incivilities occur every day. Some of the bad stuff is a reflection of a racist, culturally insensitive environment, and some of it—much of it—is *not.* Some of it merely reflects life on the wards. What is necessary is to balance that life with another life: the life of friends and family, religious institutions, bicycle rides, trashy novels, adventure movies, pets, whatever you have around you to cushion the soul. Of course, everyone needs such balance. For the medical student navigating the clinical years, however, the intensity of the training experiences and the time commitment involved make it very difficult to find time and emotional space for that other life. It is even more important, then, to carve out a little time, however brief, for the interludes that keep one emotionally balanced (see Chapter 6). Who wants to be cared for by a physician who is not fully human?

SUGGESTED READING

Carson, B., & Murphey, C. (1990). *Gifted hands: The Ben Carson story* (pp. 104-126). Grand Rapids, MI: Zondervan.

> *Although Dr. Carson's memoir does not go into detail about his clinical years as a medical student, the chapters on his postgraduate training years are descriptive of many of the experiences shared by students and house officers of color in predominantly White teaching institutions.*

Griffith, E. E. H. (1998). *Race and excellence: My dialogue with Chester Pierce* (pp. 43-45). Iowa City: University of Iowa Press.

> *These two African American psychiatrists, from two different generations, provide valuable insights derived from their experiences in a largely White professional milieu. Dr. Pierce's recollections of his clinical years as a*

medical student, although brief, serve as a poignant reminder that it is pos-
sible to achieve excellence in the face of adversity.

Klass, P. (1987). *A not entirely benign procedure: Four years as a medical
student.* New York: Putnam.

> *Klass's observations about her interactions with patients, nurses, physi-*
> *cians, and other students are funny, insightful, and instructive.*

Lightfoot, S. L. (1988). *Balm in Gilead: Journey of a healer* (pp. 178, 196-
201). Reading, MA: Addison-Wesley.

> *This biography of Margaret Morgan Lawrence, a pioneering African Amer-*
> *ican psychiatrist and educator, is based on conversations with the author,*
> *her daughter. The referenced pages deal specifically with her clinical years*
> *as a medical student, but the entire work is an inspirational account of the*
> *struggle of a woman of color to establish herself as a medical professional.*

4 Now What Will I Do?

Preparing for Residency

Carmen Webb, MD

The clinical demands during fourth year are usually far less stressful than the demands of third year. On the other hand, fourth year requires that you make choices about your future career, a process that can also generate tremendous uncertainty and enormous stress. You are expected to decide on the generalist or specialty area in which you will practice and then to choose the residency program that will provide you with your skills and shape your future attitudes toward practice for the next three to seven years. These decisions may be particularly difficult for minority students who feel responsibility to family, community, or ethnic group and must balance that responsibility with their own aspirations. The following pages will outline some tips to guide your thinking and offer suggestions about managing the process after you've made a decision. Caution: This is not meant to be an exhaustive manual for choosing and entering a residency program. There are many excellent resources (American Academy of Family Physicians, 1990; Taylor, 1986) that cover these issues. Check with your minority affairs or student affairs office.

Choosing a Specialty

Although some students settle on a specialty near the end of third year, you may very well be one of the many who are still trying to decide which one is right for you. Many studies report relationships between personal characteristics and specialty choice (Kassebaum, Szenas, & Schuchert, 1996; Taylor, 1986; Zeldow & Daugherty, 1991). Yet none of the studies are definitive for the individual. And most of this research examines the factors that determine the way students choose a specialty, not which factors determine the "right" choice. Although there is no magic set of characteristics that defines whether a particular specialty is right for a particular person, there *are* specific areas and questions to help you guide your thinking.

Guiding Questions and Issues

A Passion for the Area. Do you love the specialty area? Do you like thinking about it, hearing about it, and talking about it? Do you find yourself reading about the topic even when you don't have to?

The Way You Think. When asked why I chose psychiatry, I usually answer "because that's the way I think." When I was a medical student and heard about a patient with a gastrointestinal bleed, my first thought was how frightened the patient must have been. My second thought was "is it esophageal varices or is it an ulcer?" In other words, in a nonemergent situation, my mind goes first to the emotional, then to the physical. In what sequence does your mind naturally progress? Similarly, is your approach to problems primarily to "fix it," to examine the "why of it," or to "process it"? Knowing "the way you think" will help you to identify the specialty area that feels most natural. What is more, because you think that way most of the time, the area supporting that mode of thinking is probably the area in which you'll have the greatest aptitude.

The Culture. By now you understand what's meant by the culture of medicine (if not, see Chapter 1). Did you like the pediatrics culture? Do you like the pace of surgery? Do you like the approach of obstetrics and gynecology attendings and residents to patients? Are minorities well represented in this specialty? How important is it to you to have colleagues of your ethnicity in your field? Also, would you prefer to spend the majority of your time with doctors (pathology or radiology) or with patients (primary care)? Are you most fulfilled by treating the very ill (oncology) or by enhancing the condition of the healthier patient (plastic surgery)?

The Potential Practice Settings. Is the specialty almost certainly hospital based (anesthesiology, ER medicine, surgery), or is there a potential mix (internal medicine, psychiatry, OB-GYN). Will you need to be in a large metropolitan area near a tertiary care hospital to practice (cardiothoracic surgery)? Is a rural setting more appealing (family practice)?

The Money. How important is the money to you? Be honest with yourself if with no one else. It may be that after all the blood, sweat, and tears—and money—that you have invested in this career, you may really want a fatter purse than you once did. The satisfaction of seeing the underserved served may not be enough remuneration alone for your labor. How much do you want to make? If your specialty isn't going to provide that money, can you accept that long term? Are you willing to work more to supplement your income?

The Lifestyle. Any specialty can be incredibly demanding. It's possible to work 12-hour days, seven days a week in any area. Remember, you've been trained to expect that kind of workweek. However, you do not have to choose to continue in this lifestyle. If you decide that you want a more quiescent life, consider that some specialties can be more easily moderated than others. It's harder to find an anesthesia or surgery job with no call and with a late start in the morning, but you probably can in pediatrics, psychiatry, neurology, and pathology.

The Unacceptability. It may be that you know what specialty you prefer but don't want to accept the answer. "I want to be a pathologist, but if I do that, I'll never get the kind of respect that I would if I were a surgeon." "I want to do neurosurgery, but my marriage just can't handle another seven years of training."

Even after asking yourself these questions, you may find that you still don't know what to do. Remember that if you make a decision, you are not locked into it for the rest of your life. Many, many, many physicians change specialties, especially after the first year of training. Your path may be a little circuitous, but it does not have to dead end just because you are not sure now.

A more terrifying situation than having to choose among many specialties, is realizing that you don't *love* (and sometimes don't even *like*) anything very much. After four or more years of medical school and untold hours of study and sleepless nights, you may find that you just don't like anything. Students who feel this often experience guilt and shame. "I have this wonderful opportunity—so many have sacrificed on my behalf—so many look forward to it occurring—and I just don't want to do it."

Rita was devastated. After years of looking forward to becoming a doctor, she realized that she would finally have what she wanted: prestige and respect that accompanies the profession. She was not, however, looking forward to practicing medicine. She simply disliked patient care.

Despite the fact that graduation is only a month away, Armando is as blue as he's ever been. He has kept his focus and received honors in many courses. Unfortunately, when searching for a residency, he realized that he has never wanted to be a doctor. He has pursued this career because everyone (including himself) always expected him to pursue it. When, along the way, he had inklings that this may not be the profession for him, he put them aside, telling himself that he was just stressed or tired.

The most difficult part of the dilemma for students like Rita and Armando is that they feel trapped. "If I stop now, what else will I do?" Or "If I don't practice medicine, how will I ever repay my loans?" It is an incredible loss to realize that the majority of your academic life has been spent in pursuit of the wrong career. You will not avoid grieving. But remember that you will have choices. An M.D. can be a helpful credential in many other careers (health policy, medical administration, malpractice law, CEO of a managed care organization). If you feel you can't afford any other training because of loans, you can still choose a residency that allows as little patient care as possible.

Do not get caught up in the trap of believing you have to practice because there are so few minorities who are afforded this opportunity. (How can I throw it away?) You will contribute much more in a profession that you enjoy.

Serving

Minority physicians are more likely than nonminority physicians to serve significant numbers of patients from their own ethnic group and from low socioeconomic groups (Komaromy et al., 1996). This pattern of service has been fundamental to the provision of care to many patients of color who otherwise would not receive it. It has been a way that minority persons have cared for one another through history. Black doctors treat almost six times as many

Black patients as do other doctors, and Hispanic physicians care for almost three times as many Hispanic patients as do non-Hispanic doctors (Komaromy et al., 1996, p. 1307). The benefits are enormous. Because you are there, you will know that your people are receiving quality care. You can help them to understand their illness and to navigate the health care system. You may find it easier to stay connected with your community. Many minority patients will express satisfaction and pride in seeing a physician of their own race/ethnicity (Saha, Komaromy, Koepsell, & Bindman, 1999). They may initially be more open to you because they assume you have an understanding of their background, empathy for their needs, and personal desire that they get the care they need. They may offer you encouragement in your path. This feedback can be extremely self-affirming. It is especially important therefore to honor this trust by endeavoring to understand illness and diseases that you *don't know*, by learning about the impact of their cultural background on their health. After all, it may be tempting to pretend you understand when you really don't.

> An African American patient expressed great satisfaction on seeing that her assigned medical student, Sarah, was also African American. "I'm so glad I have a student doctor who will understand me." She offered encouragement and introduced Sarah to her family. When the patient made reference to 'Hoodoo' playing a part in her illness, Sarah, though unfamiliar with the term, was reluctant to admit it.

There are, of course, those patients who see a medical student or physician of their own background as suspect. They buy into the stereotypes of minorities that are so prevalent in majority culture ("A minority doctor couldn't possibly be as skilled as a "White" doctor." "If this doctor was really any good, why would he or she be here in this community?"). Especially if you plan to enter the setting for the gratification from your people, you may feel tremendous hurt and frustration. Your excellent care may or may not alter the patient's beliefs. However, your responsibility is to continue to provide quality care despite this lack of acceptance.

What If I Don't Want to Serve "My People"?

You may have even said it in your personal statement or your interview for medical school:

When I finish, I plan to go back to the barrio or to the projects, or to work on a reservation or to be a provider for minority patients.

At the time, without any other medical school experience, you meant it. Now you have sampled the specialties, worked on the wards, seen the clinics, the barrios, and the academic centers, and when it's all said and done, you realize that you feel like one of these students:

I don't want to work solely with or even mostly with minority patients. I want to have an even mix.

I don't want to go back to my community. I worked so hard to get out of the projects and I just don't want to go back there.

I grew up in the suburbs and there were few other Puerto Ricans there. Going back to my community wouldn't be primarily working with Puerto Ricans anyway.

I want to work primarily with cystic fibrosis patients. This illness is far more common in Whites than in African Americans. If I do it, I won't be working in my community at all.

I want to stay in academic medicine and do research in a large university hospital in my hometown. Since there are few minorities in the institution I want, I won't be serving my people.

You may not have voiced these ideas aloud, even to yourself because to many, they sound almost blasphemous. "You have gotten too 'uppidy.'" "Are you forgetting who you are or where you've come from?" "How can you have taken so much without giving back?" These comments may come from family or friends in your ethnic group or you may be saying them to yourself. They may also come from attendings, administrators, or admissions committee faculty. Majority faculty members may assume all minorities want to work with other minorities. In fact, they may justify admission of minorities solely on that basis.

Minority attendings and residents may feel you have an obligation to do this, because others, including themselves, have made sacrifices for your education. There is, of course, a basis for their concerns. Minority faculty members on the admissions committees of majority schools may have fought assiduously (and often alone) for your acceptance. Hospital-based attendings may long for some minority physicians who will accept minority patient referrals in the community. Others may have a strong desire for their people to be served and feel guilt because they have not chosen to devote their careers to this service. Some of their guilt would be assuaged if someone else met the need.

However, there is a problem with the assumption that you should provide the care for your ethnic community, wherever it may be. It presumes that because you are a member of a minority group, you are capable and desirous of treating other minority patients. Although you have certain talents and capabilities in medicine, they may not include the ones your people need. If your local ethnic community is of low income, you may not, by nature, be flexible or resourceful enough to work with institutions or people who have very few resources. Just because your skin is the same color as your patients, you are not necessarily understanding of their health care needs or of their culture. And you won't automatically care more for their needs than you would for the needs of someone else.

Remember, if you are not drawn to practicing medicine within your ethnic group, it does not mean that you cannot work effectively for or within your community. Your service to other minorities can come in the form of serving on boards, public speaking, mentoring young adults, and so on.

Minority patients deserve excellent care. They will not receive it from a physician who does not really want (or who does not have the necessary skills) to be there. The pressure you may feel from others to practice in a minority community will stem from their own beliefs, concerns, and passion. These are valid. You have a responsibility to your patients to examine your *own* beliefs, passions, and abilities. Then choose a practice setting that is a good fit for you.

Mastering the Process

The Residency Application Process:
A Brand New System

> All these years. All this time. And now I have to start that application process all over again.

It's true. You have completed applications before. But the process of applying for residency is a brand new system. It is an important system to master if you are to get the residency you want.

Where Should I Apply?

Now that I know what I am going to do, with which of the hundreds of programs do I cast my lot? Finding the best program to meet your training needs is hard enough. If you are trying to consider the needs of a family, significant other, or children, the decision-making process can be extremely difficult. Because the pile of residency brochures can be intimidating, try to digest them a little at a time. Try to read, or at least glance through them as you receive them.

You will likely get guidance from your adviser or your department of student affairs. (If you do not, ask them for it.) Remember, it is in your school's best interest for you to match[1] and especially for you to get one of your top choices. They report to potential applicants the numbers of students that match successfully. Weigh their advice thoughtfully. They will encourage you to apply to places that you have the best chance of entering and will tell you if you have a poor chance for a particular residency spot or specialty. On the other hand, suppose you have your heart set on a particular program. It is probably wise to pursue the opportunity even without a strong chance. People who discourage you from applying to some specialty may have their own agenda, not your best interest, at heart. And even if their advice is absolutely right, this may be the time that you beat the odds and match to that long-shot program.

If you have been advised (rightly or wrongly) that you will have a hard time getting into a certain program or specialty and you decide to apply anyway, put a *firm backup plan* in place. Too many times, students don't match because they have not put any safety nets down. If dermatology is a very tough specialty to get into given your grades, apply also to programs in another specialty. If California programs are in such high demand that your chances are slim, apply to more attainable programs in other states. Check out your backup plan with minority affairs, your adviser, or your mentor.

You can easily get caught up in applying everywhere, however, do *not* apply anywhere you are sure you do not want to go. Yes, you want to get a spot. But you will perform poorly if you are miserable. Fortunately, your student budget will often limit the number of applications you can submit (because you will need to have money left over for interview traveling).

The Personal Statement

You wrote a personal statement for medical school and maybe even for college. As much as you may find it difficult to express yourself honestly within the boundaries of medical culture, this task is before you—again. The personal statement is your presentation of you and your credentials. You usually begin to write this around May of your third year, which is a time when your feelings may range from excited and relieved to disillusioned and exhausted. You may not feel like giving more of yourself, even on paper. You may have armored yourself so well that you can't find any inner self to express. Give yourself permission to feel any way that you do; then take a deep breath and dig in. The first step is to do your homework. What does your specialty look for in a candidate? Some want to hear about your research in medical education; others are more interested in your breadth of clinical experience. Unlike the medical school personal statement, not all specialties frankly *care* if you are well-rounded, so ask clinical faculty members and academic deans for advice.

Most programs will be looking to see if there is anything in your character or your past history that suggests that you will have trouble working within their residency program. Of the personal challenges you have had in your medical school career, some may have had a visible affect on your performance. Consider *very* carefully if, and how, you will include them. Talk to trusted mentors about how much, if any, to include. It is usually necessary to explain any leaves of absence, but in the statement, emphasize the way the experience has helped to enhance your value to their program (e.g., you have matured from the experience).

Most programs want to know if you are really serious about their specialty. They don't want to use up a slot for someone who may choose to drop out after six months. They also want to know if you can handle the academic load. Competitive programs in particular will want to know what you will contribute to their program in the field. Unfair or not, programs usually question this most vigilantly for minority candidates. Be ready to present your academic strengths in your statement. Have several people read and critique it. (It is still true that you must perform better than your majority colleagues to get the same recognition. Unintentional grammatical errors in your statement may often be attributed to a "language problem" or "poor reading and writing skills" because of your ethnic background.)

Choose people who will give you specific feedback. Make sure that at least one of these people is knowledgeable about English grammar and syntax. Try to have your narrative reviewed by persons from majority culture, minority culture, and your specialty. The idea is not to make all their suggested changes but to help you understand how you will be received through a variety of cultural lenses. Obviously, if all these people are to give you feedback, they will need the statement well before the deadline. Write it early.

The Dean's Letter

Make an appointment to meet with your dean to discuss your dean's letter. Bring a copy of your curriculum vitae. If you are given an opportunity to read the letter, take it! You need to know what has been said about you so that you can anticipate the types of questions you'll be asked.

How important are recommendations versus personal statements versus grades versus deans' letters versus interviews versus personal phone calls from colleagues to your getting a residency? Good question. In an unpublished study, a student affairs dean (L. Hiner, personal communication, March 1997) surveyed 50 programs and learned that the importance apparently varies by specialty. However, all specialties consistently found the interview extremely important. You may get some insight about particular programs by talking to the department in your institution.

Getting Recommendations

All residency programs will require recommendations (usually two or three) from attendings who have observed your performance. At least one will need to be from attendings within your specialty. So whom should you choose? You have, of course, read Chapter 3 during third year so you have worked hard to shine on the floors. Thus, to get a recommendation, you will select from a rotation in which you did well. Preferably, pick someone who respects your work and likes you as a person. The letter writer's true feelings will come out on paper, and residency directors are good at reading between the lines.

All faculty members are busy. They do not get paid extra or get credit in their department for writing recommendations. So ask around. Find out which attendings are reliable about getting recommendations in on time. Ask to receive the recommendation long before the deadline.

Caution: There are always stories about students who thought they were well liked by an attending but received a *Milquetoast* recommendation. This often happens when the attending is just a nice man or woman and therefore is kind to every medical student, not just to you. Similarly, it's helpful to get a letter from an attending well-known in the field, but only if the recommendation is positive! Ask the attending directly: "Do you feel you can write me a strong recommendation?"

After choosing your recommenders, schedule a meeting to remind them of who you are and why you will make an excellent clinician. Provide the attending with your curriculum vitae and your personal statement. When you meet, remember that even though you are off this attending's service, the rules of the wards still apply. Dress professionally. Make sure the meeting is not on your postcall day (when you are likely to be brain dead). When they see you, they will be considering what it would be like to entrust their patients to you. Important point: You are the initiator here. If your recommender does not call you back to arrange an appointment to meet, call him or her again. If that person misses your deadline for the letter, call the next day. Get to know the secretary. He or she may help remind the attending on your behalf.

There is no way to emphasize enough the importance of getting your paperwork in on time. Early *completed* applications get considered first and most completely, before faculty and residency directors are tired of reading applications and personal statements. You may be tempted to put off asking for a recommendation, but remember, other students are not.

The Interview

In the fall of your fourth year, you will start getting invited for interviews. Waiting for these interviews can be quite exciting. What's more, because everyone is often scattered fourth year, when you meet a classmate, conversation usually centers on "so where are you interviewing?" Catching up can be fun, but if you are ambivalent about your specialty choice or haven't gotten interviews anywhere, this question will probably make you anxious. And, of course, you may occasionally have to guard against the competition game that some of your classmates will play.

> Oh, you're doing the early match for ENT? You know that's very competitive. You really think you'll get it?

> I heard only one person from our school matched to orthopedics last year. Good luck.

> You're Native American and you're a woman. You won't have any trouble getting a spot. The rest of us have had to keep our grades up though.

Ready yourself for this game. Change the subject if you don't feel like playing. If you still haven't heard from that one program in California and you need to schedule the trip to interview at the other programs in that state, you won't want to hear anything discouraging.

You will be flying, driving, and riding to many interviews this year. Do not underestimate the strain of this travel. Even for those most comfortable in the interview setting, jet lag and living out of a suitcase get old. Expect your feelings to fluctuate as you go through the year, and be aware of what you will need to maintain your positive outlook (see Chapter 6).

Try to learn about the culture of a program ahead of time, but if you have any question, assume that the rules of medical culture apply. Wear the conservative dark suit. Be absolutely on time. In fact, be early, so that you have time to catch your breath and to observe your surroundings. Many programs will arrange for you to talk with a minority resident or attending (if they have any). If no one is available, formally or informally, from your ethnic group, you probably should arrange to meet someone yourself. Be circumspect here. Some nonminority interviewers get defensive when you ask to speak with another minority person in the program.

> At the close of the interview, the residency director asked Guilda if she had any other questions. She took the opportunity to ask if there were any Latino residents whom she could contact about their experience in the program. The residency director's tone was indignant: "I can assure you that the members of this residency are not prejudiced. You will be treated like any other resident."

Interviewers may assume from your question that you suspect that they are "racist" and are trying to find out more. (In some cases, that may be true.) You may decide that if a program can't even handle your question, it may not be ready to accommodate other needs you have. But if you are interested in the program, you may simply need to ask someone else. Find out through the National Medical Association (NMA) and other organizations if there are other minority physicians affiliated with the program.

By contrast, you may be assigned exclusively to minority interviewers. This is, of course, not helpful if the program has primarily nonminority physicians and staff. You need to get a sense of what your interaction will be with colleagues day to day.

> I felt the program was trying so hard to assure me of its broad thinking and of its diversity, that I couldn't get a clear picture of the residency.

In this case, make a point to request contact with other nonminority residents or attendings.

If your interviewer is also a minority, even if he or she shares your ethnicity, be careful not to make any assumptions. Unless you have a personal relationship with that person, you do not have any reliable data about his or her beliefs, politics, or feelings about having another minority person in the program.

> One Black interviewer was insulted. The applicant, also Black, leaned back in the chair, asked him personal questions, and treated him with far less regard than any other applicant he'd previously seen (Black or non-Black). He felt that the candidate showed him certain disrespect because of their shared heritage. At best, he believed the student showed poor judgment. At worst, he wondered if the student would show him or his Black patients such disrespect later on the wards.

During the interview, you may be asked questions that are uncomfortably personal. Although state laws may vary, many questions about race, sexual preference, age, religion, national origin, or handicapped status are not illegal, especially if not used to discriminate against you. Some, however, are inappropriate. You certainly are not required to answer inappropriate questions. Yet as you know, your responses can affect your acceptance into the program. Your refusal to answer, even if done most politely, will also affect your acceptance, because it is a violation of the medical culture hierarchy. Many interviewers will not know that some questions are illegal or offensive. This is the time that your soul-searching (done ahead of time) is most helpful. Decide before you go to an interview what you are willing to disclose and what you are willing to tolerate. You may choose to give up a spot in a program if getting a slot means accepting certain questions and comments without protest.

The Decision Is Made: The Match

The National Residency Matching Program works to match residents and hospitals according to their ranking of one another. Hospitals rank applicants in the order that they want them accepted, and you rank hospitals in the order you would want to attend them. The result is that you are matched to the program that is highest on your list that has offered you a position (American

Academy of Family Physicians, 1990). Expect to feel substantial stress the week the list is due.

Finally, in March, the match results arrive. Some schools have a party, in which all results are announced; some schools give results privately. Regardless, the process can be very exciting and very stressful. It is wise to anticipate an array of feelings. You may feel terribly ambivalent. On the one hand, you may be thrilled excited, proud, and relieved to at last receive your M.D. You may feel thankful to all who have helped you through. You may feel very hopeful about your future. On the other hand, if you are leaving the city, you may be sad to leave friends or family. If you are staying in the area, you might wonder if you are missing out on opportunities elsewhere. You may also feel scared or feel regret and disappointment about ideals that you had for yourself that now won't be realized.

> Sam felt a curious letdown as he received his match results. Medical school was finally almost over. So was this all there was? All that planning and trying and hoping. He had learned a tremendous amount and had lost so many of the ideals he'd had about being a doctor. He was now very aware of his own limitations and of those of medicine.

If you have any of these feelings, try hard not to cheat yourself out of celebrating your match day and graduation. You deserve to celebrate for just getting through such rigorous training.

> I felt such a rush when I walked across the stage. I had made it! I was on my way!!!!!

Conclusion

The number of opportunities that you have ahead is both intimidating and exciting. Your willingness to be honest with yourself about your professional skills and your personal makeup are fundamental to your choosing the right medical specialty for you. Similarly, your ability to quickly gain facility with the residency selection process is critical to your finding and matching to the training program that best fits your needs. The wisdom that has brought you through medical school will sustain you through this stage as well.

NOTE

1. The "match" is a formal process "matching" students to residencies based on the preferences of both the student and the program.

REFERENCES

American Academy of Family Physicians. (1990). *A medical student's guide to strolling through the match, or, what, where, when, why, & how of residency selection.* Kansas City, MO: Author.

Cantor, J. C., Miles, E. L., Baker, L. C., & Barker, D. C. (1996). Physician service to the underserved: Implications for affirmative action in medical education. *Inquiry, 33,* 167-180.

Kassebaum, D. G., Szenas, P. L., & Schuchert, M. K. (1996). Determinants of the generalist career intentions of 1995 graduating medical students. *Academic Medicine, 71,* 197-209.

Komaromy, M., Grumach, K., Drake, M., Vranizan, K., Lurie, N., Keane, D., & Bindman, A. (1996). The role of Black and Hispanic physicians in providing health care for underserved populations. *New England Journal of Medicine, 334*(20), 1305-1310.

Saha, S., Komaromy, M., Koepsell, T., & Bindman, A. (1999). Patient-physician racial concordance and the perceived quality and use of health care. *Archives of Internal Medicine, 159,* 997-1004.

Taylor, A. D. (1986). *How to choose a medical specialty.* Philadelphia: W. B. Saunders.

Zeldow, P., & Daugherty, S. (1991). Personal profile and specialty choices of students for two medical school classes. *Academic Medicine, 66,* 283-287.

Section II
Focus on Me

Thus far, we have looked at the culture of medicine and the requirements and expectations of the four years. Now we focus on you—the person who is taking on this challenge. First we will address a question on the mind of many minority medical students: "Do I really belong here?" Then, because medical school requires that you give so much personally, we focus on how you can take care of yourself to ensure that you graduate a whole person, not just a knowledgeable automaton. Connection to family and community is a central part of the heritage of many minority students. Therefore, we explore next the ways to establish and build for yourself an additional community that is supportive and nurturing. Finally, we consider the challenges of balancing one's family and community of origin amid the pressures of medical school.

5 Do I Really Belong Here?

CARMEN WEBB, MD

You took your courses and your MCAT. You made it past the prescreening, and you underwent a grueling application process. Individual faculty members and committees reviewed your credentials. You were accepted to medical school over thousands of other applicants. However, given the nature of medical culture, you may still wonder, "Do I really belong here?" The system may not feel all that inviting. It might be completely new and different from your previous experiences or uncomfortably familiar. You may ask the question aloud to others, or you may ask it softly to yourself, so softly that you don't even realize you're asking it. "Do I, a minority student, really have a place here?" Or a corollary, " Do I, a minority student, really *deserve* to be here?"

Myths About Minorities

The origin of these questions usually has its roots in myths about minorities. These myths, like other myths, are extremely powerful. The problem with them isn't just that they sap your confidence, but that they are simply untrue.

✗ **Myth 1:** *"Minority students aren't as smart as majority students."* Some have suggested that minority students are not smart enough for medical school. Are they really bright enough to make it through all the

81

tests, not to speak of the very difficult board exams required for medical licensure? Minorities have long been believed to be less intelligent than the majority (Herrnstein & Murray, 1994). You may wonder if they are right. After all, it's their system.

The "am I smart enough" concern may be compounded for those who majored in subjects such as art, history, or English. You may look around at other students and wonder if you have the "science mind" to make it. Or you may see that you haven't had the breadth of courses others have had.

✔ **Refutation:** The problem is that this myth, even when found in print, is not accurate (Dickens, Kane, & Schultze, 1998). Intelligence is individually, not ethnically or racially, determined. Furthermore, there exist three types of intelligence, not just one: (a) componential—interpreting information in an unchanging context; (b) experiential—interpreting information in a changing context (e.g., being creative); and (c) contextual—the ability to handle the system (Sternberg, 1985, 1986). Academic performance is determined by all these types of intelligence. These as well as other personal factors are key predictors of minority performance in school (Sedlacek & Adams-Gaston, 1992; Sedlacek & Prieto, 1990; Webb et al., 1997).

✘ **Myth 2:** *"Minorities who make it through medical school are just 'slick' and have 'gotten over.' "* Even if minorities are able to break the code and understand how to make it, maybe they are just "slick." They have mastered the way to get high grades and scores, but they have not mastered the medical knowledge. One learns how to "get over" (manipulate and fool others) if faced with enough challenges in life. Maybe they have "gotten over" on their professors. Maybe they have been lucky. (And everyone knows that sooner or later your luck runs out.) Or maybe the more "liberal" teachers have taken pity on minority students, giving them passing grades when they didn't really deserve them. Or maybe they went to a prestigious undergraduate institution. The admissions committee just snapped up a "minority student from the big name school." These latter minority students have had a reputation for being "smart" for so long that people have forgotten to go back and check out their real credentials.

✔ **Refutation:** What is unclear here is that if knowing the system means you are getting over, aren't the majority students who learn the system just getting over too? You as minority students are entering a system that was not designed by minorities. The system is based on values and beliefs with origins in White Western male culture (see Chapter 1). If you are to complete your training, you must understand the system. Every student must be able to function within it—including minority students. Even when you are able to function, however, don't let anyone fool you: There is no way you could have "faked" your way through the material. There is just too much of it.

✗ **Myth 3:** *"The minority medical students you see are not qualified. They are admitted only because affirmative action laws required it."* Of those minority students admitted in the age of affirmative action, some believe that they have received "a favor" to get in. After all, that's why the system was abolished in some states, right? It gave too many advantages to unqualified people who were already receiving too many special favors.

✔ **Refutation:** This myth misses the fact that there are many minority medical students who matriculated with identical or better credentials than their majority peers. They would have met the admissions criteria with or without affirmative action. Furthermore, affirmative action simply allows admissions committees to consider race/ethnicity as a factor in admissions decisions and in targeting recruitment and educational enrichment programs. In fact, admissions committees consider many other factors *for every student* in their decisions, such as grades, test scores, maturity, interest in the field, and life experience. Race and ethnicity are now just two additional factors that admissions committees could consider. They are not passports into medical school. Affirmative action was established to remedy the long-standing discrimination against qualified minorities entering medical school. The "special favor" is a level playing field.

✗ **Myth 4:** *"Historically Black colleges don't prepare you as well as non-historically Black colleges."* The "am I smart enough?" concern may be magnified if you attended a historically Black undergraduate school. Everyone knows that these institutions are second rate and that your good grades there don't really prove anything. You are probably not as smart if you had to attend a Black college. You obviously couldn't get in anywhere else, or you would never have gone there.

✔ **Refutation:** Unfortunately, those who believe this myth rarely take time to investigate the real preparation historically Black colleges provide. They offer notable academic programs in biology, chemistry, engineering, liberal arts, and so on. Many require just as stiff admissions standards as do nonhistorically Black colleges (LaVeist & Whigham-Desir, 1999). Furthermore, many times, the self-confidence and identity development that a student may gain attending a Black college may be the exact preparation required to manage the rigors of medical school. Many students thoughtfully choose a historically Black institution because of the special opportunities for growth, the connection to one's heritage, and the excellent education.

✘ **Myth 5:** *"Minority students can't make it in medical school because they can't handle standardized tests."* Because historically, the average MCATs and board scores for minority students have been lower than those of majority students, many faculty members feel that minority students simply can't pass standardized tests. Because these types of exams are required throughout medical training and because some believe that these numbers have a direct correlation with a doctor's ability—in short, with who will become the "best doctors"—they use the statistics as a reason to deny admission to minority students.

✔ **Refutation:** Even the students who score high on the SAT or the MCAT may begin to believe the stereotype that "minority students do poorly on standardized tests" applies to them. When you hear statistics about average MCATs and GPAs of an entering medical school class, don't forget what "average means." Average means there were scores above and below. You have no idea who has the high and low scores. You may assume that "all the other students in the class" have the average GPA or that White students have the average MCAT and minority students have MCATs lower than the average. Of course, this assumption is inaccurate. Some minority students struggle with standardized exams just as some majority students do. Because the cause is often lack of experience with these exams, some students report improvement in their scores during medical school. Many other nonacademic factors may contribute to one's performance (expectation of difficulty, social support) as well (Webb, Núñez, Cohen, & Hawkins, 1996; Webb, Sedlacek, Hawkins, & Cohen, 1998; Webb, Waugh, & Herbert, 1993). There is also no research to support a *one-to-one* correlation between MCATs and later academic performance in medical school (Mitchell, 1990) or a physician's capability to provide quality patient care. Moreover, preliminary research suggests that there may be a greater correlation between clinical performance and psychosocial factors than clinical performance and test scores (Webb, Cohen, & Novack, 1997). In short, you should not hold your past scores on standardized tests or the test scores of your minority peers as evidence that you cannot pass your boards.

✗ **Myth 6:** *"Minorities who do well are trying to pretend they're better than other minorities."* Simply put, they are trying to "act White." With this myth, you may find yourself struggling with and choosing between trying to do well versus maintaining your "membership" in the group. This myth may be supported by other minorities who believe that if you achieve academically you will not maintain respect for less accomplished members of your own ethnic group. This myth may be reinforced by Whites who single you out as "the smart minority student" or "one of the good ones" or "not like other minority students."

✔ **Refutation:** The problem with this myth is that it implies that minorities by nature do not do well—and that the practice of medicine belongs only to those who are White. Minorities, of course, have not only made tremendous achievements in their countries and cultures of origin, they have overcome unspeakable challenges in this country. It is no wonder that they do well when afforded an opportunity in medicine. This book is titled "Taking My Place in Medicine" because there is a need and a role for all ethnicities throughout medicine. Although the system of training was developed by majority culture, the practice of medicine requires being with and working for patients of all cultures. Real healing requires that physicians bring their total knowledge and experience as they examine and communicate with patients of all nationalities and backgrounds. Otherwise, "conflicts and misunderstandings can result in inferior care" (Galanti, 1991, p. 1). The diversity of patients needs the knowledge and experience of a diversity of physicians (Association of American Medical Colleges, 1996).

✗ **Myth 7:** *Any care is good enough for minorities.* Students may maintain a mental picture of themselves treating other minorities. This desire is usually genuine, reflecting knowledge of substandard medical care among minorities and a desire to improve it. Some may simply enjoy working with members of their own ethnic group. However, they also may unconsciously buy into the seldom spoken but often felt sentiment that although they will never be good enough doctors to treat majority patients, they will be good enough for minority patients. This belief is perpetuated by medical culture in teaching hospitals. It is fine for trainees to "learn" on minority and low-fee patients, but only the attending physician sees private pay patients. And if you make mistakes, minority patients will forgive "one of their own." Or they will not have the resources to sue.

✔ **Refutation:** Obviously, there is a fundamental problem with this belief. Care that is not good enough for majority patients is not good enough for minority patients.

Although painful, it's important to also bear in mind that other minorities may believe these myths. They may have heard them so often that they are fooled into believing them.

Impact of the Myths

Myths about minorities need to be defined as exactly that—myths. However, your reactions to them (anger, fear, withdrawal, giving up) can be very real and will drain your energy in very real ways.

The Impostor Syndrome

The imposter syndrome is a reaction to the myths that the admissions committee did you a favor or the system made a mistake. You feel like a fraud (Morantz, Pomerleau, & Fenichel, 1982, p. 258). And you think someone is going to find out. The school will realize they made an error and maybe even kick you out. You expend time and energy to hide your deficiencies. You don't ask questions, hiding in the background so no one will know you don't know the answer. You avoid classes in which you may be called on. Obviously, this both wears on you and hides what you do know from your professors and from yourself. Even if academic deficiencies are real in some areas, this keeps you from opportunities to learn and opportunities to correct gaps in your knowledge. The impostor syndrome is deadly.

You must respond to these myths as you would any other myth. Refute them and move on. You have work to do.

Survivor Guilt

There is another reaction to the myths that may lead you to ask, "Do I belong here?" Survivor guilt. This term is most frequently used to refer to the guilt that survivors of catastrophic accidents experience (Kaplan, Sadock, & Grebb, 1994). The term is very applicable to the feelings that some high-achieving minority students have. As one student asked, "What right do I have to make it?" If your family has few resources, you are possibly among the first (sometimes the only) to go on to higher education or to have a professional career. You have reached your goal, but you look around at the rest of your family, who may still be struggling or at least are not as well off. Then the guilt comes. You may wonder if you deserve to achieve such lofty goals when no one else in your family/community/minority group has received these opportunities for employment and financial security (Davis & Watson, 1982; Spurlock, 1985). You might feel this especially if some of the family's struggles (e.g., financial) have been specifically for your achievement. Because medical school affords you no more financial resources than you had before (in fact, you probably have more debt), you can't do much to help those who are still struggling.

Even if your family has substantial resources, you may experience this guilt because others in your ethnic group are struggling. Consider this minority student:

> Tina's father owned his own business and her mother was a physician. Because the family had enough resources, she did not need financial aid, and she had a reasonable, although not unlimited, living allowance. Tina frequently gave other students rides in her car, loaned them money, and offered to pay when they grabbed dinner, even if she didn't have the time or money to do so. Soon, her grades began to suffer because of the time and energy drain of providing people transportation, and she found she did not have enough money for an important textbook one semester. When the minority affairs counselor questioned her, Tina admitted that she felt guilty that she had so many more resources than most of her African American friends.

Another kind of guilt that you may feel is derived from having to change to conform to medical culture (see Chapter 7). If your family says, "you've changed," maybe you have. They may express envy or hostility if they feel they have been left behind or perceive that *you want* to leave them behind.

The problem with the myths, the impostor syndrome, and survival guilt is that they all rob you of the opportunity to embrace your new position and, ironically, to prepare yourself to make the changes in your new community. You are so busy apologizing/hiding/feeling shame, and the like that you cannot be effective in your studies. Paradoxically, the "survivors" freeze at surviving and prevent themselves from moving on to thrive. You are not free to stretch, grow, and reach your potential.

Realistic Self-Appraisal

So how do you avoid the above pitfalls? One way is through realistic self-appraisal. This means objectively assessing your abilities and shortcomings. The concept includes taking steps to overcome any deficiencies (Tracey & Sedlacek, 1984). (It differs from academic self-assessment covered in Chapter 2, in that the latter describes an assessment of your approach to learning the material.) In medical school, realistic self-appraisal means taking stock of your situation, deciding how your knowledge base, ward performance, test-taking skills, and so on stack up and then working at maximizing the strengths and improving the areas of weakness (Webb & Núñez, 1995-1998). This ability is predictive of your academic performance, especially for minorities (Tracey & Sedlacek, 1984, 1985, 1987).

If your appraisal shows an area of strength, it's important to own that strength. Now, owning your strengths might not come naturally. You may be tempted to downplay your capabilities (it is common in this society to downplay the accomplishments of minorities). According to the myths, any of the good work you (a minority student) can manage must not be too challenging "I am doing well in microbiology, but it's no big deal. The class is easy." You may also have a tendency to discount any performance that isn't at the top of the class. You are still very good at anatomy even if someone else is better.

If realistic appraisal reveals an area of weakness, remember that accepting one's areas of weakness, "does not connote cultural or racial deficiency or inferiority" (Sedlacek & Prieto, 1990). For some, it means just accepting individual variation in ability or past effort ("I have to study physics longer to 'get it' " or "I didn't try very hard in biology"). For others, it means accepting that institutional racism is real and affects many minority students. In other words, the problem is "not a racial problem but a preparation problem." Perhaps you received an inferior education and therefore have academic deficiencies. You may have attended a school that lacks the courses or the competition required for you to build a strong academic base (Richardson, Simmons, & de los Santos, 1987). Therefore, during college you were constantly playing catch-up. Had you not been as intelligent as you are, you could not have handled it. However, you still did not make the strides ahead that some of your peers did because they were educated in a more competitive environment. The key is not to dwell on the weakness but to acknowledge it and make attempts to improve it.

OK, so how do you develop excellent realistic self-appraisal skills? There are three major steps (Webb & Núñez, 1995-1998):

1. Make an initial self-appraisal.

2. Interpret the input you get from others carefully. (Take into account the cultural lens they are using.) Maintain any valuable data. Discard the rest.

3. Manage your response.

The Initial Self-Appraisal

Try this: Take a piece of paper and as quickly as you can, write down your areas of academic excellence. You may find this difficult. Don't limit your list to areas for which you've been given awards. For example, if you have excellent analytical thinking skills, but your college didn't have a special award category for that, write it down anyway. List at least three areas.

Now, list areas that need improvement. Be careful here. Did you get a poor grade in chemistry because you're no good in it or because you do well in chemistry but do poorly in handing in assignments on time?

This list ought to be based on fact, not feelings. So list the facts. Get input from people you trust. You may now have a page that looks something like this:

Self-Appraisal (based on fact)	
Areas of Excellence	*Areas Needing Work*
Conceptual thinking skills	Memorization skills
Note writing	Presentations
Analytical thinking skills	Organizational skills
Grasp of biochemistry	Grasp of anatomy
Focused	Can at times lose the big picture

Keep this list of facts in your head, ready for immediate reference. Revise it continuously. During the clinical years, you may need to reassess and strengthen your abilities with each new rotation. This may require honing your public speaking (i.e., presentation) skills, sharpening your ability to problem solve, or improving your organizational skills. Realism recognizes the dynamic nature of self-improvement.

Interpret the Input

Now you're ready for the input that you get in medical school.

Consider a comment from an attending: "Your presentation was terrible." First, the comment was not delivered tactfully. Medical culture does not require tact in feedback, so try to disregard the way it was said (throw away the tone of voice). The blanket statement may certainly be based on some very real and specific deficiencies in your presentation. It is imperative that you find out what those are (valuable data). The blanket statement may also be based on an attending physician's feeling intimidated by your challenging his or her decisions. Although there is always room for improvement, you may have an excellent fund of knowledge and presentation ability (throw away that part of the assessment), but you will have to develop tact if you want to get a better evaluation or if you want to work effectively with other physicians in the future (valuable data).

Practice Example 1:

Sometimes the input is not so direct; take Jackie's experience:

Jackie excelled the first two years. Third year, she worked very hard, got good evaluations on her first two rotations in surgery and obstetrics/gynecology and believed she had solid clinical skills. Now, on her internal medicine rotation, her patients tell her often that they appreciate her clear treatment explanations. Yet she has begun doubting her overall abilities. Sometimes she finds that although she knows the answers to questions asked of other students on rounds, her mind goes blank when being pimped (Webb & Núñez, 1995-1998). She notices her resident not making eye contact with her. When she answers a question incorrectly, the intern rolls his eyes and suggests she go read more. When other students' err, they get a "good try." When she approaches the resident for feedback, he asks if she had to remediate anything in second year. "I know you probably got here on affirmative action, but there's no room in medicine for laziness or room temperature IQs. You should be writing more thorough notes at this point in the year and your patients need you to have the answers on the tip of your tongue."

Remember, you can miss out on some excellent information because you are too hurt, too shamed, or too angry to consider if the feedback has any real merit. To avoid this, let's examine Jackie's feedback systematically at arm's length. First, look at the factual self-appraisal. Then ask yourself if the input has origin in fact, in myths about minorities, or if it simply reflects a different cultural lens. Finally, are there any valuable data to be learned?

Self-Appraisal (based on fact)

- Fact 1: Jackie has a solid fund of knowledge. She knows the answers to most questions asked. She can explain the treatment approach to the patients.
- Fact 2: Jackie is not lazy. She works very hard on the rotations.
- Fact 3: Jackie is very bright. She catches on quickly to things and has learned the information taught in the first two years.
- Fact 4: Jackie relates well to her patients. They tell her that she is able to answer their questions.

Input Reflecting Myths About Minorities and Medical Culture Lens

Input	Myth/Medical Culture
I know you are probably here on affirmative action.	Minority students are admitted only because of affirmative action.
There is no room for laziness.	Minority students who make it through medical school are just "slick" and have gotten over. Minorities are lazy.
There is no room for room temperature IQs.	Minority students aren't as smart as majority students.

Valuable Information

Her notes may need to be written differently.

If she does not answer questions on rounds, the intern and resident will assume she doesn't know the medicine.

Plan

Because her nervousness during rounds keeps her from displaying her knowledge, she needs to work harder on this. She may also take control of the situation by providing information that she has read rather than just waiting for the next question. Perhaps she needs to practice with a fourth-year student, see a counselor, or seek out other help.

Typically, the styles of surgery and OB-GYN notes emphasize brevity, whereas medicine notes are more detailed. She needs to learn how to write a medicine-style note. Again, a fourth-year student may be able to help.

Not all input is so blatantly unkind. Some feedback may feel innocuous but still require realistic self-appraisal.

Practice Example 2:   *Someone says to you, "You are too intense!"*

Self-Appraisal (based on fact)

You are focused and persistent.
Now hold it up to different types of lenses.

Input Reflecting Different Lenses

Input	Lens
"You are too intense!"	Classmate lens: "Your ability to focus makes me nervous and I wonder if I'm studying enough." or "I'm worried that you'll get better grades/evaluations than I will."
"You are too intense!"	Family/significant other lens: "I want more of your time and attention. I wish you were more available."

Valuable Information

Others recognize that you are focused and persistent. Classmates and friends want something from you. If you are stressed, others are picking up on it, and it makes some of them uncomfortable.

Because of how painful or confusing some messages may be, it's prudent to do some external checks. Sometimes, there is *no* valuable data in the comment. Get another opinion (from someone who is objective) about how you are performing. But use caution. In this medical culture, professors and attendings become "godlike" elders or parents. Because we live in the culture every day, we may automatically seek external checks from the very people giving the messages. To decide who is best suited to give you that reality check, *look for someone with nothing to lose personally if you succeed or fail.* For example, to understand what the specific problems are in your write-up, talk to a fourth-year student or to a resident with whom you are on friendly terms. If possible, he or she should not be on our service and should not in any way be evaluating you. Is your minority affairs system in your corner? Is there a minority faculty member who is safe? If you are in a majority institution, is there a majority attending or resident or upper year who will be honest with you about how others see you? Caution: Be careful about "opening up" to those who may not be circumspect about telling your business to colleagues.

> One administrator was very supportive of minority students and in fact took pride in his willingness to be so. However, the person also felt free to "share" any private information with other faculty members "so that we can help 'those' students." This administrator was not so open with information about nonminorities. Moral: Always check out your confidantes.

Identify "safe" people. Ask around to find out if they have a proven track record with other minority students. If there is no one in your institution, make a point to get on the phone and find minority faculty members elsewhere. The National Medical Association (NMA) has a mentoring program for minority medical students. Also check for local societies of minority physicians in your area.

Manage Your Response

Many minorities have developed an external armor borne of a heritage of dealing with racism. So when you are attacked (or at least feel attacked) you may don an unreadable, blank expression. You may take on a "don't mess with me or I'll hurt you" tone. You may look down and melt. Some of these have been adaptive in other settings but may not be entirely transferable to medical culture. For instance, looking down and melting translates "weakness"— a cultural "no-no." Or a "don't mess with me" tone may translate "hostile" or "unstable" in some specialties, This may be especially true for males, if your colleagues believe the media's portrayal of minority males being "angry." Be ready to adapt the face of your armor to the right armor of protection in medical school. A calm professional tone and demeanor usually works.

When you are used to walking around with your armor on for such a long time, you may forget to take it off at night when you're alone or on your own territory. But the only way to examine input realistically *is* to remove the armor. Remind yourself of who you really are, not who you are for the attending. Remember where your real strengths lie, and identify the areas that could use some improvement. Only then should you look at the feedback.

Conclusion

Hopefully, it is now clear to you that you do belong here. The new culture of medicine, the myths, survival guilt all may lead you to believe that you don't have a place in medicine. In fact, you do. Your continued realistic appraisal of your performance and recognition of the need to adapt to the culture and refute the myths will help you to avoid letting these divert your focus. You have a right to be in medicine. Medicine needs what you will bring.

REFERENCES

Association of American Medical Colleges, Health Professionals for Diversity Coalition. (1996). *Statement from Jordan J. Cohen, M.D., President, Association of American Medical Colleges.* www.aamc.org/about/progemph/diverse/newsmkrs.htm

Davis, G., & Watson, G. (1982). *Black life in corporate America.* Garden City, NY: Anchor/Doubleday.

Dickens, W. T., Kane, T. J., & Schultze, C. L. (1998). *Does the bell curve ring true?* Washington, DC: Brookings Institution.

Galanti, G.-A. (1991). *Caring for patients from different cultures.* Philadelphia: University of Pennsylvania Press.

Herrnstein, R. J., & Murray, C. (1994). *The bell curve: Intelligence and class structure in American life.* New York: Free Press.

Kaplan, H. I., Sadock, B. J., & Grebb, J. A. (1994). *Kaplan and Sadock's synopsis of psychiatry.* Baltimore: Williams & Wilkins.

LaVeist, T., & Whigham-Desir, M. (1999, January). The 50 best colleges for African Americans. *Black Enterprise, 29,* 71-82.

Mitchell, K. (1990). Traditional predictors of performance in medical school. *Academic Medicine, 65,* 149-158.

Morantz, R., Pomerleau, C., & Fenichel, C. (1982). *In her own words: Oral histories of women physicians. New Haven, CT: Yale University Press.*

Richardson, R. C., Simmons, H., & De los Santos, A. G. (1987, May/June). Graduating minority students lessons from ten success stories. *Change,* pp. 20-27.

Sedlacek, W. E., & Adams-Gaston, J. (1992). Predicting the academic success of student-athletes using SAT and noncognitive variables. *Journal of Counseling & Development, 70*(6), 724-727.

Sedlacek, W. E., & Prieto, D. O. (1990). Predicting minority students' success in medical school. *Academic Medicine, 65*(3), 161-166.

Spurlock, J. (1985). Survival guilt and the Afro-American of achievement. *Journal of the National Medical Association, 77*(1), 29-32.

Sternberg, R. J. (1985). *Beyond IQ.* London: Cambridge University Press.

Sternberg, R. J. (1986). What would better intelligence tests look like? In *Measures in the college admissions process* (pp. 146-150). New York: College Entrance Examination Board.

Tracey, T. J., & Sedlacek, W. E. (1984). Noncognitive variables in predicting academic success by race. *Measurement and Evaluation in Guidance, 16,* 171-178.

Tracey, T. J., & Sedlacek, W. E. (1985). The relationship of noncognitive variables to academic success: A longitudinal comparison by race. *Journal of College Student Personnel, 26,* 405-410.

Tracey, T. J., & Sedlacek, W. E. (1987). Prediction of college graduation using noncognitive variables by race. *Measurement and Evaluation in Counseling and Development, 19*(4), 177-184.

Webb, C., Cohen, D., & Novack, D. (1997, November). *Beyond academics: Predicting clinical skills.* Paper presented at the Association of American Medical Colleges Annual Meeting, Washington, DC.

Webb, C., & Núñez, A. (1995-1998). Non-cognitive tools. In A. Núñez & C. Webb (Eds.), *Navigating the medical culture: Medical student course curricular document.* Philadelphia: MCP Hahnemann University.

Webb, C., Núñez, A., Cohen, D., & Hawkins, M. (1996, November). *Noncognitive variables: From analysis to intervention.* Paper presented to the Research Forum of the Group on Student Affairs—Minority

Affairs Section at the Association of American Medical Colleges Annual Meeting, San Francisco.

Webb, C. T., Sedlacek, W., Cohen, D., Shields, P., Gracely, E., Hawkins, M., & Nieman, L. (1997). The impact of nonacademic variables on performance at two medical schools. *Journal of the National Medical Association, 89*(3), 173-180.

Webb, C., Sedlacek, W., Hawkins, M., & Cohen, D. (1998, November). *Using noncognitive characteristics to predict USMLE step I scores.* Paper presented at the Association of American Medical Colleges Annual Meeting, New Orleans, LA.

Webb, C., Waugh, F., & Herbert, J. (1993). Predictors of Black students' board performance: MCATs are not the whole story *Academic Medicine, 68,* 204-205.

6 Taking Care of Myself

CARMEN WEBB, MD

Because you have read it or because you are now living it, the fact that medical school makes considerable demands should now be obvious. Your training requires that you give yourself fully in the service of caring for others. What may not be obvious is how you are supposed to find the time and energy to take care of yourself. This chapter addresses the many facets of self-care: understanding your needs, evaluating your supports, finding personal renewal, coping with stress and, if needed, seeking mental health care.

Taking Stock

Martia is tired. Very tired. She has always been the one on whom everybody in her family depends. During college, she worked full-time, acted as a second mother to her younger siblings (cooking, cleaning, disciplining), helped pay tuition to a special school for her disabled cousin, volunteered at the Salvation Army, and directed the church choir. During medical school, she continued to carry her home responsibilities, although she did give up the Salvation Army and the choir. She has received honors in most courses and is proud of her ability to handle so many challenges without calling on others for support. Now, however, she feels very stressed. Her grandmother has been diagnosed with cancer, her youngest sibling has run away from home, and she has just learned that she did not get honors in the rotation for her desired specialty. She has always handled things before—worse things—and cannot figure out why she is having such a hard time now.

Martia approached the stresses in her life as she always had—by just taking them in stride. That worked for awhile. But everyone has limits. Had Martia recognized her needs before, she might have sought support before life became overwhelming.

Medical school requires a tremendous amount of time, energy, and stamina. You will need to be sure that your own needs are met if you are going to keep up with the pace. And because it is virtually impossible to handle everything yourself, even the most able student will need support of some kind over the four years. That is difficult for those who see themselves as always able to take care of themselves or who have been the ones to take care of others. If you evaluate your needs and your supports beforehand, you will have far more control in crisis situations.

Understanding My Needs

The best assurance that you'll get appropriate support is to know what you need.

Just as cars need gas, oil, and washing for routine maintenance, we need different types of support to keep our lives running smoothly. Your needs probably fall into five general areas: time, life maintenance, emotional/social support, concrete advice, and spiritual support (Stein, 1990).

Evaluate Your Needs in These Areas

Time. "Do this for me so I will have more time." "I just need time to be by myself."

If there is one thing that every medical student needs, it's time (Webb & Núñez, 1995-1998). Consider: How much more time do you need? Actually take a minute now to calculate the time you need for studying, maintenance, socializing, and so on. How many hours do you need in a day?

Life Maintenance (meals, laundry, cleaning, paying bills, etc.). How much time, money, and physical stamina does it take each week to maintain your body and your shelter? Are any of the tasks relaxing? Which take the most out of you?

Emotional/Social Needs. "I want to vent about medical school." "I want to talk about things unrelated to medical school." "I need someone with whom to work out/go dancing/go to a movie."

Showing vulnerability may or may not be acceptable for your gender in your culture. It may be that expressing emotion is all right but asking for support for it is not (i.e., people will listen, but respond with "just be strong"). Whether or not asking for emotional support is acceptable, you will undoubtedly need to do it at some point. How often could you use an ear? You will also need some recreation and social outlet. What kinds of social interaction (activities, types of people) do you need? How often do you need them? How much of an outlet you need may be related to how much enjoyment you already get from interacting with peers at school.

Concrete Advice. "I need to understand the medical school system better." "Do I have to do research to get into that specialty?" "Do I really need to buy that textbook?"

You will find that there is information you just won't have unless someone imparts it to you. And there are suggestions and advice related to your rotations, your patient care decisions, and your colleagues that you would be foolish to refuse. Seeking this advice is an important means of survival. What sources for that advice do you already have? What do you need to add?

Spiritual Needs. "I need a place to meditate." " I need to find a group that worships like I do."

During medical school, many students feel the need to connect with something larger than themselves. Even if you have never practiced any form of organized religion or worship before, you may find yourself seeking strength in your spirit. What places, people, time, and so on do you need to maintain your spiritual self?

Find and Evaluate Your Supports to Meet Your Needs

After you've determined what you need, the next step is to get those needs met. However we aren't cars, so we can't just go to the local garage for service. We need to map out our options for getting support in those areas.

As you think through the above list of needs, ask, "How do I get these needs met now?" "Who are the people (family, friends, mentors) and what are the groups (religious groups, clubs) and activities (dance, music, computer games) that support me?" Are they available? What items on the list remain uncovered? Then ask, "Given the supports I have, how *effective* are they?" When you evaluate, consider *high-maintenance support, pseudosupport,* and *misguided support.*

High-Maintenance Support

How much time and energy does it take to maintain your support system?

When Nicole has a problem, she often talks to her classmate Sherry. However, Sherry also uses Nicole for a sounding board and tends to spend long periods struggling with life decisions. Sometimes Nicole finds she has spent hours on the telephone dealing with Sherry's problems.

Juan's father contributes generously to his living expenses. However, his father feels that he has a major say in Juan's decisions (whether or not he needs more clothes, whether he should be studying or going out with friends Friday night, etc.).

These students both have willing supporters, but they must invest considerable time or emotional energy to sustain their supports.

Pseudosupport

There are supporters who are probably more aptly called pseudosupporters. They gladly offer help but subtly put you down for asking. "I knew medical school would be too much for you." Or "You can't handle it—sure I'll do it." This group is important to identify early. Waste no time asking or worrying about their responses. Take the request elsewhere.

Misguided Support

Knowing the kind of support that you do need is as important as knowing the kind of support that you don't. For example, consider Marie:

Marie's family, who lives two hours away, has always encouraged and supported her goal. All her younger siblings and cousins look up to her. The first week of medical school, her great aunt who had been like a second mother, called to say she had broken her arm. Marie drove down to provide support. When Marie had a birthday the weekend before the first biochemistry test, her whole family drove up for the weekend to celebrate because she couldn't go home. After failing the test, Marie knew she needed more study time, so she began to stay up till 1 a.m. every night. Her family members, also concerned, each began to call her the night before any test to let her know they were thinking of her (Webb & Núñez, 1995-1998).

Marie finds her family offering all kinds of support, in the form that they always have: their presence. Unfortunately, this is not the kind of support she needs the week before exams.

Now you have evaluated your supports. Do you have adequate support to get all your needs met? What or whom do you need to add? Jot remaining needs down, as well as how you plan to obtain support for them. Tap family, friends, community, minority affairs, other school resources, or faculty members (in any area). *If you feel you will have difficulty finding your support, evaluate the obstacles.*

Evaluate the Obstacles to Getting Support to Meet Your Needs

The primary block to your getting the support that you need may be *the way that you see yourself.* You may feel shame—"I should be able to support myself"—as though being on the receiving end is the equivalent of weakness. If your role in life has been as a caretaker, it may be very difficult to see yourself as anything else. Or you may feel guilt: "People have given me so much/ worked so hard to help me get to this point. How can I ask for more?" The problem with all these responses is that they are beside the point. The point is the task at hand—getting through medical school with a sense of well-being. And you don't have the time or the luxury to allow these feelings to prevent your needs from being met. A related block is *your reluctance to say no to supporters.* Marie's ever-present family (above) will know how to support Marie (allow her to be unavailable) only if she tells them how—probably more than once. In this case, saying "no" is as important as "please will you do this." ("No, I can't talk on the phone tonight." "No, I don't want you to come see me because I need to study.")

A parallel situation occurs with friends—and more subtly with medical school friends. Because you are "going through the war together," your class-mates often become your closest confidants. This may be a real dilemma in the minority community if you empathize with one another's challenges; you may be tempted to give more than is academically healthy for you— particularly if you have made a pact to "get one another through." You may sacrifice self for your medical student friends.

Clearly, it's difficult to say, "No I don't have time to get together." Even if you can bring yourself to do so, you may waste as much time feeling guilty or worried about losing the relationship as you would have spent getting together. So one possible approach is to turn on your answering machine and turn the volume way down. This eliminates having to say "no" over and over. Let your family and friends know what you are doing so they won't panic when they can't reach you for days on end. Another way to become unavail-able is to simply change your location. Exam week is probably a bad time to sit in the library amid anxious peers. Finding a new study spot that's tempo-rarily inaccessible may be helpful.

Because many of you, especially as minority medical students, have been in the supporter role for some time, you may find it impossible and even undesir-able to stop supporting others. The key here is limit setting. When is it time to say "no" to the request to see the family or to help a friend? Sometimes the support will take too much time and will compromise your academic progress or stress you out so much that you can't study. When do you make excep-tions? As a rule of thumb, ask yourself this question:

Is supporting _____ *in this way more important than getting good grades/passing this test in medical school?*

Another obstacle to getting support may be *others*. If you do finally ask for support, you may be turned down. The problem is that others may not be accustomed to thinking of you as needing help. They may be uncomfortable with the idea of your asking, given your previous role, and may not anticipate your needs. Therefore, from the beginning, be as honest as you can about the challenges of medical school and about how they are affecting you. Further-more, it is crucial to be specific when you ask for help. Not "I miss you honey" but "Would you please spend Tuesday with me?" Not "I just don't have any time" but "Would you go grocery shopping for me during exam week?" Others may simply be uncomfortable with the request itself. It may be too time-consuming, costly, or emotionally charged (e.g., "listen to me vent about medical school, but just listen. Don't offer me solutions or try to fix it"). There are also those who may agree to your requests but may not always be willing or able to accommodate our needs. After it's been so difficult to ask, this may come as a major blow (no matter why they refuse). A backup plan ("if mom says no, I'll ask my friend") is good to have at this point. Not only will it provide a way to meet the need, but it will decrease the sense of distress that you may feel when turned down. Always take a moment to consider alternatives before you ask.

Making a Plan

Finding Renewal

Even if your supports are in place and life is running pretty smoothly, remember that a car that's running fine still needs regular service. Similarly, humans need regular maintenance to maintain their emotional, intellectual, social, spiritual, and physical stamina. All these parts are tapped during medical school and all of them need renewal.

> John spent all day in the OR. His feet were tired and his arms were aching from holding a retractor for 5 hours. He was mentally exhausted from trying to call up little factoids from first and second year regarding the anatomy, nerves, and blood supply of the pelvis. Mostly though, he was spent from trying to hold back his anger and to hold on to his academic self-esteem while the surgeon berated him whenever he did not know an answer. He had held on simply by praying for strength all day. All John can think of now is getting home and falling into bed.

John's ordeal is not atypical. The challenges of medical school exhaust us. Obviously, he needs sleep, but John also needs to replenish his emotional, intellectual, social, spiritual, and physical stamina.

Emotional Renewal

What energizes you emotionally? What gives your mood a boost? Is it encouragement? Is it finishing a project? Is it praise? Maybe it's spending time with people to whom you feel connected. Or maybe you've noticed the positive effect of sunshine.

You might be taught to sweep your feelings and emotions under the rug (Halpern, 1993) in medical culture (see Chapter 1). Certainly, you learn not to let them show. It is in fact considered almost adaptive to build an armor that ignores your feelings ("Just let it roll off your back. If your resident asks you how you're doing, say you are doing fine," one student was advised by the rest of the minority students). If it is in your nature or cultural background to express your emotions, you will find this practice stifling. Furthermore, you have to be aware of your emotions if you are going to address them (Arlow, 1989).

Some students find that journaling, the process of recording their thoughts, allows them to express and examine their feelings. Others find talking to a counselor or therapist helpful. For many, creativity is another way to express their emotions. Unfortunately, if you used to paint, draw, or play an instrument, you may have stopped in medical school. As some have said, "I don't want to do it if I can't do it right." But dust off your tools. You need what the music or color or art can give to you. Move your focus away from your skill and toward your personal expression. If you found renewal through dance or movement, "create" a way to do that now. Get a friend to dance with you. Draw posters for an AIDS benefit. Play the piano in the student lounge.

> ▶ I was friendly with a resident, and one day we shared some pretty personal things. I felt great at the time, but afterward he treated me with condescension on the wards.
>
> ▶ I was so exhausted after studying for the last phase of exams. I went out with a woman I met at a club. We had what I thought was a simple night of fun, with no obligations. It turns out she wanted much more. I feel bad because I know I really hurt her.
>
> ▶ I had been on call every third night for four weeks. I felt so wasted and unattractive. One particular evening, one of the physician assistants on the floors hit on me and I took him up on it. Now I've learned that he is HIV positive.

Intimacy feeds many of us emotionally. You may find it through a very honest, personal conversation. If you find it through a sexual relationship, be careful. As your need for intimacy increases, and your time and opportunity to express it decreases, you will be very tempted to choose *any* relationship to meet your needs. The problem with "instant" physical or emotional intimacy (besides health risks) is that it causes a greater energy drain in the long run. The people you hook up with are still people. Usually, they will want something back. Be careful how you share yourself when you are trying to get emotionally charged.

Social Renewal

While in medical school, it is common to feel "out of touch" at times. You miss dates with friends and the latest movies, and you don't always hear about world events. Renewal includes reestablishing social contact. Maintaining these connections is covered in Chapter 7, "Building a Community."

Intellectual Renewal

Your mental muscles are likely being stretched and exercised daily, particularly in the first two years. But your desire for intellectual stimulation is not limited to biological science. You may also thrive on English literature, political science, music, or other areas that challenge your mind. The most effective way to feed this mental need is through regular doses of nonmedical input. Whether it is public radio on the way to school, a sci-fi novel, or trivia games with nonmedical family/friends, you will benefit from the interlude. Granted, you may not be able to contribute new insights to the discussion, but you will get the minimum monthly requirement of intellectual renewal.

Spiritual Renewal

For many minority students, a spiritual life is a key source of peace and empowerment. The role of spirituality in the heritages of African American (Mbiti, 1991; Raboteau, 1978), Puerto Rican (Garcia-Preto, 1982), Mexican American (Elizondo, 1988), and Native American (Oren Lyons, 1990) people is great. And many of us carry our heritage with us, whether or not we practice any organized religion. However, the spiritual self is sometimes the easiest to ignore. Medical culture encourages you to "suck it up" and go on. "Don't look too hard at the inside of yourself, at your inner workings; just keep working." Depending on the culture of your medical school, your spiritual beliefs may or may not be shared. Spiritual renewal requires introspection and self-awareness. And that requires time and space.

You may find that spiritual health comes through more informal and private times of renewal with meditation, prayer, nature, private study of scripture, and the like. However, even if you live alone, books and lecture notes can crowd out time for spiritual renewal. Double that if you have a roommate. Triple it if you have a spouse, or partner, or children. Decide how you will maintain the public and/or private time. Something will have to go. Not this.

If you enjoy participating in a worship service, communal prayer time, or Bible class, you may struggle to make time to attend. You could be tempted to simply give up on participating in a formal religious community, especially if your faith supports a personal spiritual connection. Yet some faith communities provide an extended family. They offer support and encouragement, social activities, and opportunities to build leadership and creative talents (Felton, 1980; Griffith, Young, & Smith, 1984). Much of your world, especially the first two years, consists of people between the ages of 21 and 40. You may need the nurture of an elder and contact with a wider range of people to experience a more complete perspective and community. The privation of these connections may prove a substantial loss. Therefore, if a religious community has been important to you, try to establish some form of this now.

> ▶ One group of students who attend a historically Black medical school agreed that spiritual life is extremely important to "making it." Said one, "There are no atheists in medical school."
>
> ▶ A student from a majority school that had no other medical students from her island lamented that she was unable to find other students with whom she could talk about her faith. She found that others just didn't understand her form of worship.

Be creative in your search for a spiritual resting place. One group of Mexican American medical students gained access to a place of private meditation in a Jesuit sanctuary. One Island student visited her religious community several miles away once a month and worshiped at the local church other weeks. It was just enough to keep her going. A group of minority students decided to start a study of Biblical figures who sustained themselves through difficult work. Your school may have groups to support certain types of fellowship (e.g., Christian Medical and Dental Society, Muslim Student Association). And so on. Do not be stymied by the extent to which your options fall short of your preferred religious community. Instead, consider the most important elements of your faith family and look for a body that provides at least some of these elements.

Creating new ways to look inside at your spiritual self will be necessary. You can't leave this part of yourself alone for four years. You need the energy and power.

Physical Renewal

On the most basic level, physical renewal is good for you. Exercise helps you to relax and to stay strong and physically vital. Several students testify that it provides a rush and sense of well-being.

> I run approximately 45 minutes every day after class. It helps me shake the troubles of the day.

> I used to roller skate around the lake or study in the park to break the monotony of memorizing. Now I'm in a medical school downtown and don't have that.

If you moved from a mild climate to attend a medical school located in a colder area, then biking/walking/jogging/surfing can be out of the question six months out of the year. Countless students have found themselves frustrated without their usual method of exercise. The key is to build a new plan for exercise into your new life. Even if exercise is among your least favorite activities, try to weave it into your daily routine. Especially if you are usually sitting (as during your first and second year), try to do one thing each day. Walk to school if feasible; take the steps (not the elevator); park further away. In addition, choose some form of exercise that is enjoyable, for 30 minutes over the course of the day, something to which you can look forward (Nivins, 1998; Rippe, 1999). One student started walking with a classmate during lunchtime or after school. It was a good motivator and helped her connect with someone. Another student found that kickboxing was an excellent way to reduce stress.

Designing Personalized Methods of Coping With Stress

Unless your car stays in the garage, it will encounter rain, snow, sun, dirt, and so on. Weatherizing your vehicle protects it from elements. Similarly, preparing for stress helps you to cope with life's inevitable challenges. Of course, if you are thinking, "I don't get stressed," check your pulse. Stress is a function of being alive. It has been defined as the "mental and physical changes when demands are made on us to adapt and change" (Belfer, 1989, p. 109). By the time you matriculate, you undoubtedly have coped with intense stress—the premedical courses, the MCAT, the interviews, the waiting for an acceptance letter—in addition to (for many) significant stress from life events alone. But the coping styles that you've used up until now to get here don't necessarily work for medical school life. In medical school, change and stress are a way of life. The overwhelming studies, the limited exposure to life out-side medical school, the postponement of many life events (in terms of income, relationships, etc.)—each of these is stressful by itself. However, now all are occurring at the same time. Plus, these stressors are ongoing. Plus those people who might normally support you may not have experienced medical school and therefore can not understand what you are going through. As a minority student, you may experience more stress than your nonminority colleagues (Anderson, 1991). Minority students report greater sense of their lives being out of their control after just one year of medical school (Pyskoty, Richman, & Flaherty, 1990). Additional options, steps to take when you feel stress, are needed. Without new options, we will automatically turn to old coping styles. Then when they don't work, we may try to use them over and over, longer, and more intensely. We keep coping the same way because that's all we know.

Examples of What Worked Before That May Not Work Now	
Procrastination for several days	Escape for several days
Demanding change	Sticking with the same game plan even though it isn't really working
Talking to classmates the night before a test (they may not have time/may not understand)	Focusing long-term on other ful-filling activities (community work, others' problems)
Handling things on your own	Giving up sleeping/eating

Although stress is unavoidable, it can either cripple us or energize us. The way you choose to cope with stress determines its impact on your life (Folkman & Lazarus, 1980; Linn & Zeppa, 1984). When someone's heart stops, the emergency room doctor can't afford to get stuck in the horror of the moment but must automatically turn to specific steps to help the patient. Simi-larly, you will do well to have specific, *effective* steps to deal with stress. We need both: (a) prophylaxis—prevention of the stress we know is coming and then (b) intervention—a healthy method of dealing with stress when it does come.

Prophylaxis: Prevention of the Stress We Know Is Coming (Webb & Núñez, 1995-1998). Recognize when you are stressed. This may sound obvious, but we don't necessarily think about our personal signs of stress. Do a self-check after a situation that is stressful for most people (a big test, a loss, illness, etc.), even if you don't feel stressed. Ask yourself "What are the ways I usually know that I'm stressed?"

- *Make a body check.* Check yourself for physical signs of stress that everyone recognizes (trembling, increased heart rate, dry mouth, sweating) and less obvious signs (diarrhea, fidgeting).
- *Make a mind check.* Are you trying not to think about the thing? Are you telling yourself you are incapable, stupid, incompetent, and so on? Do you feel numb?
- *Do a behavior check.* Are you drinking/eating/smoking more? Are you drugging? Are you watching a lot of TV? Are you losing yourself for days in your novels? Are you skipping showers?
- *Do an environment check.* Is your house a mess (or extremely clean)? Do you have laundry piled to the roof, or is your sock drawer arranged by color and size?

Recognizing your stress response puts you in control. It allows you to get on top of the stress early.

Intervention: Healthy Methods of Dealing With Stress When It Comes. So what do you do when you recognize your stress?

♦ First, make a speedy assessment. Run through the body, mind, emotion, behavior, and environment checks for signs of stress. Are there lots of signs? Do I need to act now? If so, try to address the physical things that contribute to the tension. Unclench your fists. Take some slow deep breaths. Put down the ice cream or the beer. You may feel immediately uncomfortable, but try to stick it out.

♦ Second, what is at stake? What am I most afraid will happen? Be complete, looking at both the positive and the negative. Is the concern realistic? Your assessment of what's at stake is closely related to your stress level (Folkman & Lazarus, 1980). For example, Am I really likely to fail this exam? I have studied so little that I have a very good chance of failing. But I also have a chance of passing it. Is my best friend really going to disown me for not being in touch? He or she will be mad but probably won't stop being my friend.

♦ Third, ask yourself: Can I honestly change the situation? There is no point in beating your head against a brick wall. By the same token, you cheat yourself if you sit paralyzed while you hold the power to change something. Appraisal of how changeable a situation is, is related to how much burden you experience from a problem (Solomon & Draine, 1995a, 1995b).

If the Situation Can Be Changed

If the situation can be changed, list some plausible ways *you* can effect the change: "Studying more increases my chances of passing." "Going to the professor will help me understand this better." Then stop and count the cost. What will the price of making the change be? Is the price worth it? For instance, is passing my exam worth swallowing my pride and asking for a tutor?

OK, let's say the change is worth it. Then make a plan. What exactly will you do? Call to make an appointment with the dean. Go to minority affairs and solicit their advocacy. Ask that person you don't know very well, but who knows the stuff cold, to study with you.

If Change Is Not Possible

If there is no plausible way to change the situation, or if the plan is not worth the cost, it's most effective to stop trying to fix the problem and focus on helping yourself feel less stressed.

♦ In the midst of the situation, you can't see all sides. An outside perspective from a professor, upperclassman, or someone like that (carefully chosen!) can help you stay focused on what is really important. For example, ask a physician if a patient ever asked if he or she repeated a year in medical school or how many times he or she took the boards. Ask a resident, "Will this biochemistry exam keep me from getting a surgery residency?" Then consider changing your own perspective. "If I have to repeat the year, is my life really over?" Some repeaters say that they had a chance to learn more and to become better doctors.

♦ Reduce your discomfort. Plan limited healthy escapes. The key words are *plan* and *limited.* Long-term escape and avoidance of problems are never useful solutions. They usually lead to facing a bigger mess later. But if you limit your escapes (reading a short story, watching a half-hour of a *good* sitcom, eating *one* ice-cream cone), you can relieve stress. If you doubt your willpower to limit the escapes, plan to have someone call you at the end of your TV show, or plan to meet a study partner at a certain time. *Word to the wise:* Alcohol and drugs are never good options for relieving stress. They may help you escape short-term, but they will lead to serious problems (see below).

Increase your relaxation time. Do *not* eliminate your time to take care of yourself. If you haven't scheduled break time, do it now (at least 30 minutes a day for pleasure; see Chapter 2, "Balance"). If you have breaks, increase them from 30-minutes to 45 minutes. During that time, do the things you know to be helpful. Don't give in to the temptation to punish yourself for not achieving what you hoped or for making mistakes. Do things that you know will be comforting to you (a bubble bath, prayer, talk with a good friend, exercise). This is not the time, though, to do things that are "good for you" but not satisfying. For example, exercise is important and can relieve stress, but it belongs in the 30-minute period only if you enjoy the *process* of exercise, not just the result.

Another option is to get up. Go do something. Stop the "Oh my gosh, what if ____ happens?" cycle. Stop thinking about the problem for the moment. Remind yourself of your value as a person and of why you are here; you are becoming a physician.

A Word About the Worst Way to Cope

One of the worst ways you can cope is to use alcohol and/or drugs to escape from stress and to manage sleep deprivation. Medical students reportedly use alcohol and tranquilizers more than their nonmedical student peers do (Conard, Hughes, Baldwin, Achenbach, & Sheehan, 1988); 23% of medical students are heavy drinkers, 12% use marijuana or other drugs regularly, and 5% report dependence on psychoactive drugs (Clarke, Eckenfels, Daugherty, & Fawcett, 1987; Maddux, Hoppe, & Costello, 1986; McAuliffe et al., 1986; Schwartz, Lewis, Hoffman, & Kyriazi, 1990). The few studies of minority medical students show that Black students used drugs less frequently than majority students (Forney, Forney, Fischer, & Richards, 1988), but Black physicians are more likely to abuse tranquilizers than any other drug (Carter, 1989).

You will learn a great deal in the classroom about substance use, but there may be little discussion about your vulnerability to it as a student. The myth, even among faculty and administrators, is that substance abuse is not prevalent in *their* institution. However, you will see those around you, majority and minority students, drinking way too much, smoking or growing pot, or downing cocaine, uppers, tranquilizers, and other drugs. Some will steal drugs from the medication cart or operating room. Often, many students and residents will see this happening but say nothing. As in other "families," physicians do not wish to admit to themselves, to one another, and certainly not to the outside world that someone "in the family," could have such a dangerous, embarrassing, or illegal problem. Furthermore, the usual social taboos against confronting others with their substance use are magnified in medical culture. We fear damaging a colleague's career (as though the substance is not doing far more damage). It's certainly easier to tell yourself that the drinking and drugging will "stop in the third year" or "end after graduation." Yet for training residents and practicing physicians, stress and sleep deprivation and therefore the risk of substance abuse grow greater as training progresses. And not dealing with drug/alcohol use can lead to poor judgment, medical mistakes, and patient harm. If you hesitate to address impairment in yourself or someone else, consider whether you want a preventable patient mistreatment on your conscience.

If you have any questions about the role alcohol/drugs play in your life, meet for a consultation with a psychiatrist or an addictions counselor. Because substance abuse and addiction are illnesses, addressing them means getting treatment, not punishment. All medical schools are required to have some venue to address student impairment. Some are better developed than others. Find out (in your student handbook or from an adviser you trust) the kind of help your school offers. You want a program that is confidential, that is oriented to treatment (not just to monitoring), and that provides ongoing support. You also want an advocate to help minimize any potential negative impact on your schooling. If the institution's program is inadequate, don't hesitate to identify treatment outside. Find a local Alcohol Anonymous, Narcotic Anonymous, or Cocaine Anonymous group in your phone book, go to a meeting, and start identifying other resources from there.

Bottom line: You have a far better chance of minimizing the impact of substances on your finances, career, and family if *you* are the one to initiate treatment.

Reasons to Get Mental Health Care

Sometimes, even the best methods of handling stress may be insufficient. Many students who have had no difficulty handling previous challenges may be distressed and simply confused when they begin to have emotional difficulties in medical school. "How could this happen to me?" Because medical students do not lose their status as human beings when they enter the physician culture, they are not inoculated against emotional problems. Students still have mental illnesses before, during, and after matriculating. Although more serious illness may have eliminated many students from the admissions process, mental illnesses common in the general population affect medical students as well (major depressive disorder, anxiety disorder, bipolar disorder, obsessive compulsive disorder, alcohol/drug-related disorders, and eating disorders). The rates for medical students are higher in some cases than in the general population (Dickstein, Stephenson, & Hinz, 1990). It is wise to buy personal disability insurance now, *before* you need it.

Finding Mental Health Support

Reasons You May Hesitate to Get Mental Health Care

- I don't need it because I'm not crazy.
- My fellow medical students will find out.
- It will go in my permanent academic record.
- My family will find out.
- It is against my cultural values.
- It costs too much.
- I should be able to handle things on my own.

Reasons You May Hesitate to Get Care

Yet the layperson's (and maybe your) belief is that medical students and physicians cannot suffer mental illness, perhaps because to many, the need for mental health care means, "you're crazy." Television and movie images come to mind of severely ill, poorly functioning, or violent persons. This belief is magnified within medical culture where physicians are "strong" and "conquer illness." (Although intellectually aware that doctors can get sick, deep down physicians may not believe it can really happen to them.) The false stigma of mental illness may prevent you—now in a group at high risk—from seeking care.

Other concerns about getting care are quite valid (Myers, 1997). You certainly do *not* want any record of your health history, physical or mental, on your academic record. You want your clerkship evaluations and applications to residency evaluated on the basis of academic ability, not someone's fears about your health status. Your health care information should be revealed at your discretion only.

You may have particular apprehension about entering the mental health system as a minority person. Many minority groups have not fared well in the health care system in general, and the mental health care system is no exception. Historically, we have been misdiagnosed (Airhihenbuwa, 1995; Davis & Proctor, 1989; Garb, 1997). Psychotherapy has been financially unobtainable and minorities in lower-socioeconomic groups have been thought poor candidates for psychotherapy. Higher-income minorities have been mistakenly considered to be "just like nonminorities, only a different color." These experiences have simply compounded the history of distrust many minority groups have toward psychiatry. However, today, there is excellent, culturally competent care available in most all communities.

Choosing the Right Help

The solution is to seek out the right place and person to provide care. The most accessible choice may be the school's student counseling or mental health service. The advantage of using this service is that the provider will likely be used to working with medical students and familiar with the pressures you are under. That person may even be familiar with the professors and attendings you encounter. Importantly, he or she will not be overly impressed with or judgmental of your "status" as a doctor-to-be. If you choose to get care in the community, the advantage is that it provides greater choice and greater anonymity with respect to school personnel. You may need to do more legwork to find someone, however. In both settings, therapists should agree to maintain confidentiality unless you give written consent to release any records. Because all health care costs money, you may use your insurance. Many worry that this will start a paper trail that will hurt them in their future careers. The insurance companies do have access to your health records but can release no information without your consent. Although some hospitals and residency applications ask about past health care, this fact cannot stand in the way of getting help; the benefits far outweigh the risks. Bottom line: Poor quality of life, poor grades, poor relationships or illness left untreated are far more likely to affect your career than a paper trail.

Whom would I see? If you are having considerable difficulty managing things day to day or you find yourself extremely unhappy for no reason that is clear to you, I recommend that your first checkup be done by a psychiatrist. This will ensure a thorough evaluation. (Is your lack of motivation simply run of the mill, or is there evidence of underlying depression, hypothyroidism, or other physiological cause?) The person to see for treatment depends on the problem. Psychiatrists who offer both therapy and/or medication treatment are your best bet, because they provide the best integration of care and the benefit of one-stop-shopping. Otherwise, a primary care doctor (if he or she is well versed in psychiatric illness) can help with medication and a psychologist or social worker can conduct ongoing therapy.

Important Questions to Ask Personnel in the School-Based System

▶ Are my records ever, under any circumstances, released to anyone such as my family, the dean, the professors or the promotions committees?

▶ Am I ever likely to be evaluated by this person during medical school? Is this person a course director, a clerkship director, an attending I can't avoid on the wards? (Someone who just teaches but doesn't evaluate is probably OK).

▶ Is the office a reasonable distance from the main flow of classmate and faculty traffic?

Now here's another question. *Am I best served by choosing a therapist who is a member of my minority group?* There has been a great deal of literature addressing this issue (Atkinson, Poston, Furlong, & Mercado, 1989; Cooper & Lesser, 1997; Lago & Thompson, 1996; Sue & Sue, 1977). Certainly, another minority has experienced similar challenges of not being in the majority in this country and may have a better chance of understanding you. But bear in mind that "minorities" represent a very heterogeneous group with varied life experiences. The most important criteria is that the person you see is committed to understanding your personal culture as it affects your experience. Your therapist should not assume that your culture is like his or her own or like the culture of other minorities he or she has known (or read about or seen on TV). Finally, remember that there are many types of therapy. Your therapy should be appropriate to your needs or diagnosis. Ask the therapist to describe the treatment and why it's important for your issues.

Conclusion

Although medicine offers fulfilling and satisfying opportunities, at times, it can also exact a tremendous toll on your personal resources. To continue to grow and enjoy life both personally and professionally, you do well to make as strong a commitment to taking care of yourself as you do to taking care of your patients.

REFERENCES

Airhihenbuwa, C. O. (1995). *Health and culture beyond the Western paradigm.* Thousand Oaks, CA: Sage.

Anderson, L. P. (1991). Acculturative stress: A theory of relevance to Black Americans. *Clinical Psychology Review, 11,* 685-702.

Arlow, J. A. (1989). Psychoanalysis. In R. J. Corsini & D. Wedding (Eds.), *Current psychotherapies* (pp. 29-62). Itasca, IL: F. E. Peacock.

Atkinson, D. R., Poston, W. C., Furlong, M. J., & Mercado, P. (1989). Ethnic group preferences for counselor characteristics. *Journal of Counseling Psychology, 36*(1), 68-72.

Belfer, B. (1989). Stress and the medical practitioner. *Stress Medicine, 5,* 109-113.

Carter, J. H. (1989). Impaired Black physicians: A methodology for detection and rehabilitation. *Journal of the National Medical Association, 81*(6), 663-667.

Clark, D. C., Eckenfels, E. J., Daugherty, S. R., & Fawcett, J. (1987). Alcohol-use patterns through medical school. *Journal of the American Medical Association, 257,* 2921-2926.

Conard, S., Hughes, P., Baldwin, D., Achenbach, K., & Sheehan, D. V. (1988). Substance use by fourth year students at 13 U.S. medical schools. *Journal of Medical Education, 63*(10), 747-758.

Cooper, M., & Lesser, J. (1997). How race affects the helping process: A case of cross racial therapy. *Clinical Social Work Journal, 25*(3), 323-335.

Davis, L. E., & Proctor, E. K. (1989). *Race, gender and class.* Englewood Cliffs, NJ: Prentice Hall.

Dickstein, L. J., Stephenson, J. J., & Hinz, L. D. (1990). Psychiatric impairment in medical students. *Academic Medicine, 65,* 588-593.

Elizondo, V. (1988). *The future is Mestizo.* Oak Park, IL: Meyer Stones.

Felton, J. C. M. (1980). *The care of souls in the Black church.* New York: Martin Luther King Fellow's Press.

Folkman, S., & Lazarus, R. S. (1980). An analysis of coping in the middle-aged community sample. *Journal of Health and Social Behavior, 21,* 219-239.

Forney, P., Forney, M., Fischer, P., & Richards, J. (1988). Sociocultural correlates of substance use among medical students. *Journal of Drug Education, 18*(2), 97-108.

Garb, H. N. (1997). Race bias, social class bias, and gender bias in clinical judgment. *Clinical Psychology-Science & Practice, 4*(2), 99-120.

Garcia-Preto, N. (1982). Puerto Rican families. In M. McGoldrick, J. Pearce, & J. Giordano (Eds.), *Ethnicity and family therapy* (pp. 164-185). New York: Guilford.

Griffith, E., Young, J. L., & Smith, D. L. (1984). An analysis of the therapeutic elements in a Black church service. *Hospital and Community Psychiatry, 35*(5), 464-469.

Halpern, J. (1993). Empathy: Using resonance emotions in the service of curiosity. In H. Spiro, M. M. Curnen, E. Peschel, & D. S. James (Eds.), *Empathy and the practice of medicine* (pp. 166-167). New Haven, CT: Yale University Press.

Lago, C., & Thompson, J. (1996). *Race, culture and counselling.* Buckingham, UK: Open University Press.

Linn, B. S., & Zeppa, R. (1984). Stress in junior medical students: Relationship to personality and performance. *Journal of Medical Education, 59,* 7-12.

Maddux, J., Hoppe, S., & Costello, R. (1986). Psychoactive substance use among medical students. *American Journal of Psychiatry, 143,* 187-191.

Mbiti, J. S. (1969). *African religions and philosophy.* Portsmouth, NH: Heinemann Education Publishers.

Mbiti, J. S. (1991). *Introduction to African Religion.* Oxford, UK: Heinemann Educational Publishers.

McAuliffe, W. E., Rohman, M., Santangelo, S., Feldman, B., Magnuson, E., Sobol, A., & Weissman, J. (1986). Risk factors of drug impairment in random samples of physicians and medical students. *International Journal of the Addictions, 22,* 825-841.

Myers, M. F. (1997). Management of medical students' health problems. *Advances in Psychiatric Treatment, 3,* 259-266.

Nivins, B. (1998). *Success strategies for African Americans.* New York: Plume.

Oren Lyons, O. (1990). Wisdomkeepers: Meetings with Native American spiritual elders. In S. Wall & H. Arden (Eds.), *The earthsong collection.* Hillsboro, OR: Beyond Words.

Pyskoty, C. E., Richman, J. A., & Flaherty, J. A. (1990). Psychosocial assets and mental health of minority medical students. *Academic Medicine, 65*(9), 581-585.

Raboteau, A. (1978). *Slave religion.* Oxford, UK: Oxford University Press.

Rippe, J. (1999, July 15). How to stay fit, how not to overdo it: The basics. *Bottom Line/Personal.* (Search for Rippe at www.blp.net)

Schwartz, R., Lewis, D. C., Hoffman, N. G., & Kyriazi, M. (1990). Cocaine and marijuana use by medical students before and during medical school. *Archives of Internal Medicine, 150,* 883-886.

Solomon, P., & Draine, J. (1995a). Adaptive coping among family members of persons with serious mental illness. *Psychiatric Services, 46*(11), 1156-1160.

Solomon, P., & Draine, J. (1995b). Subjective burden among family members of mentally ill adults: Relation to stress, coping and adaptation. *American Journal of Orthopsychiatry, 65*(3), 419-427.

Stein, H. F. (1990). *American medicine as culture.* Boulder, CO: Westview.

Sue, D. W., & Sue, D. (1977). Barriers to effective cross-cultural counseling. *Journal of Counseling Psychology, 24*(5), 420-429.

Webb, C., & Núñez, A. (1995-1998). Non-cognitive tools. In A. Núñez & C. Webb (Eds.), *Navigating the medical culture: Medical student course curricular document.* Philadelphia, PA: MCP Hahnemann University.

7 Building a Community

CARMEN WEBB, MD
GEORGE C. GARDINER, MD

Loneliness is one of the most common problems medical students face. For some, it starts the first day. You look around at a sea of faces and see no one from your home community. Or you see the same people you competed furiously against during premed or postbaccalaureate programs. The personal drain on you as a student makes a community that can offer support, connection, and resources all the more necessary. Therefore, in medical school, it is critical to build your own community.

The Problem: Isolation

I have lots of acquaintances here but no real friends.

It seems like no one has time to hang out together and really talk.

We complain about medical school, but that's the closest we get to real feelings.

I'm from the area, but I'm at school so much that I feel out of touch with my family and community.

I am just plain lonely.

Some students find that the connections that began during orientation may not grow as much as they had hoped when school starts. Everyone is relatively friendly and relaxed during the get-to-know-you socials and introductory picnics. But come that first day of classes, people get *very* focused. You may study together, but folks are willing to spend far less time playing ball or going shopping or talking late into the night.

> I made wonderful friends while in medical school—some White, one from Pakistan. But I longed to talk with someone who was Mexican American. I missed talking to someone without having to explain the nuances of my heritage or language.

If you have a live-in partner and/or children, your loneliness may be different. Your medical school friends may spend lots of time in the library studying together. You try to rush home after class to maximize time with your family. And maybe family members cannot relate to medical school, or you feel your friends don't understand what it's like to have to juggle both home and school. No one seems to understand just what it's like for *you.*

For minority students in majority institutions, the loneliness may be compounded. If there is no central meeting area for minority students, such as the Office of Minority Affairs, students may not naturally run into each other. And if busy with school, they may not take time to make connections. Even if your primary friends are not minority students, you may miss contact with other minority students once in a while.

For some, the isolation may be self-imposed. You may withdraw when stressed or focused. If you are having academic difficulty, you may find yourself declining social activities because you know you must study—or because you are ashamed.

> Laurie was devastated when she learned that she would have to repeat the year. She had kept her academic problems pretty much to herself, so no one really knew she was even at-risk. She dreaded seeing people from her class, fearing she'd have to tell them the truth. She started just studying at home and going to lab on the weekends.

The danger of isolation is that it generates more isolation. Everyone is busy, and no one has a lot of time to come track you down. And if you constantly turn people down, they eventually quit asking. You feel more lonely and left out, and you avoid people more. Friends don't know how you feel, so they can't help you.

Isolation results from not connecting with people. To mitigate the isolation, you need a community—people with whom you share beliefs, feelings, political views, outlooks, history, or heritage. And because most students don't necessarily find a ready-made community, build it you must.

com•mu•ni•ty (kə-myōō′nĭ-tē) *noun*
1) A group of people living in the same locality. 2) A group of people having common interests. 3) a. Similarity or identity: *a community of interests.* b. Sharing, participation, and fellowship. (*American Heritage Dictionary of the English Language,* 3rd ed., 1992)

Choosing My Crowd

While in medical school, your community may be composed of a brand new group of medical students, family and old friends (if any are nearby), and/or nonmedical people in your institution or city. Whoever is included, you need to feel comfortable with this group and have in common with them some values and interests that are fundamental to the person you are. You need them to care about you and to be available. You'll want them to be tolerant of your regression and unavailability during the most stressful times. This is true for all students. However, there are particular issues for minority students in choosing a crowd, especially if they seek to build their community among other minority students.

> We started out with three Puerto Rican students in a class of over 200. Our medical school was not very welcoming to Puerto Ricans. By the end of the first year, we were down to two. The two of us left lamented together, feeling extremely vulnerable. "What are we going to do," I asked despairingly. "Well," came the reply, "we stick together like white on rice."

If you are at a majority school and there are few minority students, you may find that the group is relatively close-knit and sticks together. Similarly, if your particular ethnicity is not well represented among the other minorities, your group may also become very tight. Regardless, your goal is to stay close for comfort and strength through difficult circumstances. Not uncommonly, the group makes a pact that they will pull together and make sure that everyone graduates. For example, if a student gets an old exam, he or she makes certain that everyone has access to a copy. If you have a central minority affairs or Student National Medical Association (SNMA) office, you may even have a collection of old notes, tests, and useful textbooks from past years. You notice if someone is missing from class and make a point to look for that person to make sure everything is OK. Upper-year students may offer invaluable guidance to those coming after about the best ways to study for a certain class, the expectations of some ward attendings, and so on. They may also offer just plain medical knowledge.

> Before the first day of introduction to clinical medicine, an upper year got together we seven minority students and went over the physical exam with us. The next day on the wards, we were golden!

This sense of drawing together is not limited to small numbers of minority students at majority schools. Students at one historically Black medical school said, "It feels like a family here." One student said that she felt that both peers and faculty looked out for her, cared about her, and noticed if she was gone. There was the spirit of a shared history and goals. You may receive criticism at majority schools from people who see a group of Blacks or Hispanics or Native Americans "always together." Certainly, others who share nonracial similarities are just as cohesive (Tatum, 1997); your skin color simply makes your assembly more visible. Some have suggested that the criticism comes from those who feel threatened by a group of minorities who, if joined together, might "do them harm." Or perhaps the naysayers feel left out or rejected. Regardless, if the community feels comfortable, embrace it. Pulling together, sharing resources, with the elders helping the younger, are strategies that have allowed many minority groups to thrive in this country (Felton, 1980). There is no need to apologize for this positive coping strategy (Tatum, 1997). And rest assured that others are choosing their communities without asking for your approval.

Still, the dynamics of the minority community can vary widely depending on the school, on the year of study, and on the number of minority students in attendance. Sometimes in larger minority student populations, cliques form and people do not always get along. Because of your greater numbers, students may feel less committed to "sticking together" to make it through. Unfortunately, some minority students have wasted precious time fighting among themselves when they could be drawing support from one another. Such conflicts have resulted in academic disaster. If you have any role in continuing the conflict, *let it go.* Your being right is far less important than your medical degree. Similarly, if you hear about such a conflict, encourage the parties to reach resolution, but immediately move the conversation on. Do not get drawn in. Even if you are trying to help, you can lose many hours acting as peacemaker. If necessary, a trusted adviser or minority affairs director can act as mediator.

If you gravitate toward a racially or ethnically homogeneous group, it is wise to make it your home base, not your exclusive affiliation. You're likely to miss wonderful friendships if you neglect the wider community. From an academic perspective, you will need the resources of the collegewide academic, professional, and social activities. If you become an active participant in the total medical school experience, you will have access to valuable knowledge and information (old exams, information about informal reviews by the professor, and any number of other key resources). When it comes time for your recommendations, or if you run into any problems, you will want to be known by both majority and minority administration and faculty members. If people know you, they are more likely to advocate for you. It is much better to have this scenario in the promotions committee:

> "Oh, Melinda had some trouble in microbiology, but she's a good student. We needn't worry about her."

Rather than,

> "Oh, another minority student failed the microbiology exam. Maybe she should repeat the course."

Well, what if your main group of friends are not those in your ethnic group? If your school has a number of minority students of any size, you may be expected to make them your primary community. You may also be expected to depend on the Department of Minority Affairs as your primary support system. If you don't "hang," the other students may interpret that as your rejecting them or as your "not knowing who you are."

- There are only a few of us here. Seems like she'd want to stick together.
- He must think he's White. Wait till he gets to the wards. Then he'll realize who his real friends are.

But what if you don't feel you have anything in common with the other Black, Mexican American, Puerto Rican, or Native American students? After all, just because you are all minorities, doesn't mean you share all (or any) experiences. It certainly doesn't ensure that you will like each other.

> I am from an island where my parents are landowners, physicians, and lawyers themselves. I came over here for medical school. I found the other Black people here had a victim mentality and were hung up on needing to prove themselves. I don't feel I need to prove anything. I just could not relate to them. I had more in common with the White students.

> The minority students usually sat together in the right middle section of the lecture hall. I liked to sit in the front and had gotten friendly with the people (nonminorities) who also sat there. We formed a study group, and I just never got to know the other minority students as well. At orientation, we had all been encouraged to stick together. I felt tremendous obligation to spend my time with the other students of color. You know, I just didn't need that kind of pressure in the middle of trying to keep up with everything else.

Advice to these students parallels the advice given to those who *do* wish a close connection with other minorities. Do not cut yourself off. Some find that the support they enjoyed the first two years is just not there in the clinical years. Friends are scattered, and the attendings may see you as simply "another minority student." You will likely need the support and guidance of other minority students who have already made it through. Try to find a way to stay affiliated at least to some degree with the group. Make a point to attend SNMA or Boricua/Latino Health Organization (BLHO) meetings once a month, or bring a dish to the Cinco de Mayo celebration. Of course, in some cases, the group will not accept you at all if your main group of friends is outside. In this instance, you simply have to choose the community that is the best fit for you.

Word of Caution: In the new medical school community, you run the risk of taking on the same degree of community involvement that gave you so much success and gratification in undergraduate school. This may present an opportunity to stay involved in an old, successful activity while avoiding the distressing new job of being a medical student. All too often, this "retreat to the familiar" has a negative effect on academic performance. For a few students, initial academic stumbling sometimes results in an even greater involvement in community-type activities to avoid academic issues, thereby, setting up a downward spiral. A similar dilemma may emerge with the family in your community (see below).

Finding a Religious Community

For some, a very important source of their community is the people with whom they share religious beliefs, worship and/or meditation experiences. That is, a religious community. This is covered in chapter 6. Do *not* neglect this area.

The Role of the Office of Minority Affairs in My Community

Your school, if it is a majority institution, may have a department of minority affairs. This office is designed to assist students, as one school describes, "in academic and personal adjustment to medical school, [to] provide support and assistance, academic and personal counseling, and organize and implement special events and activities which encourage the identification of support systems within the minority community" (MCP Hahnemann University, 1998). The office can become the center, both physically and symbolically, of the minority community. It may become the gathering place. It may be the hub for notices of everything from the location of the next SNMA meeting to the date of the postexam party. You may find the old exam file there or the list of recent graduates in the specialty you want.

> I failed biochemistry, and I got a letter from the Minority Support Services. But I avoided going because I was so embarrassed. After all, I was supposed to be the shining star. I had gotten an academic scholarship because of my good record. I felt I had let everyone down.

You can expect the office to keep up with your academic progress. You may get a note from them if you do especially well on an exam or if your grades begin to drop. If they call you in, go. The office will make suggestions about potential supports or changes in strategies you might use. Some students make the mistake of assuming that the office is only for students having trouble. Not so. Retention means not just surviving but also thriving. As the director gets to know you, he or she may recommend you for special awards or scholarships. You may be asked to sit on medical school committees or be recommended for consideration for research opportunities. When important transition points come up, this office may arrange to have a group of upper years give insights about life on the wards, studying for the boards, or choosing a residency. It may help you prepare your personal statement or point you in the right direction for financial help. Promotions and admissions committees may look to it for guidance on the fate of minority students. It is extremely important that you check out this potential resource. This office may have a great impact on your future.

The Department of Minority Affairs will have a reputation among students in terms of how helpful, accessible, and safe it is. Will the people in it protect your confidences? Will they advocate for you with the administration? Do they have any power? No matter the reputation, you need to determine its role in your community for yourself. Be aware that the institution may abdicate all its responsibility for support of minority students to this department. (If you have an academic problem, substance abuse problem, a need for financial aid, etc., the dean expects the Office of Minority Affairs to take care of it.) The problem? This expectation is not always matched by adequate resources or personnel, putting the office in a terrible position. If there is one director and one secretary for 100 minority students, there is no way to build recruitment, admission, retention, and career advising effectively. In fact, this is really a setup for failure, causing frustration for everyone. The administration wants to know why so many students are having trouble if they are spending money on the Office of Minority Affairs. The director feels overwhelmed and pulled in 50 directions. And the students feel adrift if they are told that this is their main resource.

- *The director is hired to look out for the minorities here, but when I go to talk to her, she's always in a meeting.*
- *The office isn't doing nearly enough to deal with that professor who made a crack about "questioning your minority patients in particular about drug use."*

Your frustration is compounded when you share the image of the director and staff as elders or parental figures. You may find that you feel very disappointed, even betrayed. Particularly if there were many "elders" from your own community who are now far away, the people in this office may be the closest you have to parental figures. The bottom line here is to avoid writing off your office as a resource if it doesn't meet all your expectations and needs. If not effective advocates, are they good listeners? If they are not very warm, can they help you to locate minority physicians in the area? Do they have information on preparation programs for the boards? Finally, even if you deem the office completely useless for you, check in every once in awhile. You never know when you may need someone there to know you.

If you are in a majority institution that does not have support services for minority students, what can you do? At the point when you know the lay of the land, bring that absence to the attention of the dean. A letter from whatever minority presence there is, and a request for a meeting with the dean to discuss your concerns, is a reasonable first step. However, in the meantime, identify some physician support yourself. Consider asking minority faculty members (if there are any) for help. In one school, a minority faculty member[1] met with the minority students every week in a classroom for one hour at noon, just to offer support, suggestions, and a presence. His consistent attendance served as a central meeting point for both upper- and lower-year students. If a faculty member isn't available, try to identify a minority physician in the community. This physician will likely be less able to provide advice on negotiating the system of the institution, but he or she could be, again, a nidus of hope.

Finding Mentors
in My Community

Another very important person to build into your community is a mentor. It is quite possible that as a minority student, you have accomplished your goals without the help of anyone in the medical field. If so, you may wonder if you really need a mentor. It's a legitimate question. You could probably make it through medical school without one. But the advantage of having a mentor is your opportunity to enhance your performance in the classroom and in the hospital setting, to progress more readily, and to have more pleasure in your work (Grady, 1991; Wright & Wright, 1987).

So What Is a Mentor? "A mentor is more than a role model—one who sets an example. A mentor is someone who actively participates in your personal and/or professional development" (Grady, 1991, p. 8). The ideal mentor is one "who will not rest until you succeed."[2]

What Can a Mentor Do for You (Grady, 1991; Wright & Wright, 1987)? First, a mentor will provide information. On the most basic level, he or she can tell you what is expected of you on the wards, what residency training is like, and how to apply for a scholarship. *Second,* a mentor may be crucial in helping you to fully realize your abilities and in giving you an honest assessment of your skills. It's quite likely that you have not had the breadth of experience needed to recognize your talent for scientific writing or your fine teaching abilities. Your mentor may invite you to shadow him or her during office hours or ask you to present with him or her at a research conference. Often, students have spent the majority of their adult lives working or preparing for medical school and have not had time to investigate the myriad options. *Third,* many minorities have been told of their deficiencies so often that they no longer value their abilities. Others are aware of their abilities but believe they will not be valued in the professional arena. Your mentor will help you to develop a realistic self-appraisal—to assess your own performance (see Chapter 5). You may need the encouragement (or strong-arming) to motivate you to go out and pursue, or even simply accept, challenges. Said one African American woman, "Only with my mentor's insistence did I agree to present my first paper. Even as I made the promise, I was thinking of how ludicrous the idea was!" *Fourth,* a mentor can help you in networking—including you in intellectual discussions with peers, introducing you to key people, "treating you as an equal in professional organizations" (Wright & Wright, 1987). This is particularly important for the minority female who must overcome both racial and gender barriers to be taken seriously as a colleague. *Fifth,* your mentor might also introduce you to both current and historical role models. Often, schools and environments do not lend themselves to studies of such leaders in or outside of the medical field. The sheer number of historical figures alone can be encouraging. *Finally,* your mentor may be supportive to you personally. If your mentor likes and respects you as a person, he or she may help you to weather the storms of professional life. You especially want someone who will aid you in moving ahead on your career path and support you even when you are unsure and unfocused.

How Do You Find a Mentor? In most instances the storybook example of a mentor and protégé just happening on each other, "clicking," and working together happily ever after is very rare. Most likely, you will need to work on the relationship.

If you are attending a historically Black medical school, you may have an advantage in the mentoring department. In focus groups held at one such institution, African American and non-African American students alike denied any difficulty identifying mentors both within and outside of the school. They found them in classes, in administration, on the wards, and in the community.

In some institutions, you may have a mentoring program set up by your school or minority affairs office. In addition, the National Minority Mentor Recruitment Network (Grady, 1991) provides mentors for minority students. If you are one of few minorities in a majority institution, you will probably need to initiate a connection. The few faculty members of color are most likely stretched to the limit. Check with your director of minority affairs regarding who may be open to a mentoring relationship (ask for a list). Of course, if you do run into any minority residents or faculty members (in class or on the wards), make a point to introduce yourself. Some relationships begin while asking about a test question or solving a patient problem. Ask if you can sit down to discuss your career goals, their specialty, common research interests, or how that person made it through medical school. Ask if you can round with him or her one day.

Remember that no one person can fulfill all your mentoring needs. (What one person is a great researcher, teacher, advocate, clinician, networker, listener, etc.?) Therefore, you will likely have a number of mentors.

> My first real mentor was a minority faculty member who was an excellent listener and helped me negotiate the medical school culture. The summer after my first year, I met a Caucasian Ph.D. who began to guide me in the fundamentals of research. Toward the end of my fourth year, I met a minority physician who encouraged me in my desired specialty. All of them have been extremely valuable to me.

Seek mentors among both minorities and nonminorities, physicians and nonphysicians. If someone has a genuine interest in supporting your development, do not rule him or her out or in because of race or M.D. status.

In all cases, take the initiative. Don't wait for your potential mentor to call on you. You call him or her. Respectfully ask to fit into that person's schedule. However, no matter how thirsty for mentoring you are, resist the urge, like one who finds water in the desert, to start out asking a great deal of the mentor's time. These people have lives as well and may decline to help if overwhelmed by your initial requests.

Evaluating a Mentoring Relationship. Beware of detrimental mentoring relationships. You are not assisted if the mentor "helps you to death" (P. Shields, personal communication, May 1990). If your mentor feels sorry for the huge burdens you bear and decreases his or her expectations of you, you gain nothing. Although the burden is often real, pity does little to enhance your self-esteem. Neither does condescension. We can all sense when someone feels sorry for us versus empathizing with and respecting us.

Here are some other signs of an unhealthy mentoring relationship (Wright & Wright, 1987):

> A woman in my institution offered to mentor me. She was kind and protective. I realized there was a problem when she brought me to a meeting and introduced me as "her baby."

- Someone who uses you to further his or her own career. Is the person encouraging you to do a great deal of work without giving you credit for your efforts?
- Someone who rejects you personally if you do not accept opportunities he or she has to offer.
- Someone who does not support you if your opinions differ.
- Someone who pursues a romantic or sexual relationship with you.

The Family in Your Community: A Balancing Act

It's often difficult to determine the role of family in your new community. Whether your family means to you parents and children or includes also uncles, cousins, grandparents, and special friends, family is fundamental to who we are. In minority groups especially, family has traditionally played a central role in the individual's life. Our families get us started in life, providing us with direction and meaning, nurture, mutual support, and opportunities to measure and experience our own self-worth. Ideally, they give us a supply of positive memories of loving relationships. In meeting life's challenges, the relationships offer us opportunities for some very meaningful achievement and sustain us through difficult times. Even if your family relationships have been rocky, your family has provided the basis for your personal culture. Minority students who are successful academically and emotionally have learned to balance a demanding curriculum with family ties.

Autonomy Versus Family Loyalty

To survive and flourish in a hostile racial environment, many families will pull together and present a united front to the outside world. Over many generations, this strategy has been quite successful and very important to minority families. However, it may not work well when you need to move out into another part of society (i.e., medical school) and to take on a lifestyle that is different from that of your nuclear family. Family members may feel jealousy or resentment if they view your achievement as rejection, abandonment, or a reminder that they have not achieved as much. The acquisition of a *new style,* one different from your family's, can be viewed as evidence that you're no longer loyal to your family.

Time Versus Old Roles

Nurturing family members who have had a powerful influence on your development may inadvertently place demands on you to give them more time. For example, you can be very loving in response to your parents' devotion and, in fact, be very dependent on them for nurturance, guidance, and approval. This reciprocal love your parents receive may become so important that the most pressing thing for them is to continue receiving it. They might seek ways to maintain closeness, expecting you to go to school close to home, stay in frequent contact, be home every weekend, and/or stay involved in all family discussions or squabbles.

> Marco came from a small, tightly knit family. He worked in the family business throughout college. He chose a medical school near home and experienced tremendous pressure from his parents to continue his weekend work schedule. They saw his new commitment as evidence that he no longer cared about them. Only through talks with a faculty adviser were they able to slowly understand that his different role didn't mean his emotional link to them was any weaker.

Your altruism (the quality that attracted you to medicine in the first place) may cause you guilt if you are not there for your family members when they need you. If your new role as medical student is not entirely comfortable, you may gain some comfort and satisfaction from reverting to previously successful roles—that is, continuing as a pillar of support for the family.

Remaining overinvolved with the family is a trap because you need to devote considerable physical and emotional energy to the job of being a student. An overinvolved family can make it difficult to make that shift. If you or your family is unwilling or unable to "loosen up," the result is a virtual tug-of-war with tension, anxiety, guilt feelings, anger, or other uncomfortable emotional states.

Living for Your Parents

Your parents may well experience quite a bit of satisfaction in feeling their love appreciated or their guidance reinforced when you choose a particular career pathway. It is no secret that parents frequently find even more pleasure in having their children either follow in their own footsteps or achieve goals that they themselves only hoped for. This kind of vicarious enjoyment often works well for all concerned, but it can sometimes distort your parents' vision or impair their judgment. Your parents may be *overly* committed to seeing you follow a particular, prescribed direction. If carried to an extreme, it can result in your choosing a major part of your goals for their benefit.

Striking a Balance

On the one hand, you must avoid the extreme of being overly involved with your family; on the other hand, you often cannot risk total estrangement from them. This balancing act may be difficult to maintain. Learning medicine is your primary job for the next four years. So be honest with yourself about how much time and energy that requires. Accept the fact that it is necessary for you to take on a different role in your family and that you must sacrifice somewhere. Be ready for mixed feelings, such as guilt, pain, and relief, about losing those old roles and their benefits (feeling needed/connected, knowing the family news, having some control over events). Your need to redefine yourself is a natural phenomenon that all of us have experienced in medical school. You're not alone. Seek perspective from those who've been through it.

When you have thought it through, examine with your loved ones what it is that they expect and what you can anticipate *before* you encounter bumps in the road. They may have creative options. You might do your laundry while you visit; you'll attend family dinner once a month; you'll call home once a week. Remember: You may need to have this discussion several times to allow them (and you) an opportunity to get used to the changes. If necessary, engage the help of medical school staff or faculty to help family members understand that this is a temporary but absolutely necessary change. If after all your efforts, your family is still unwilling or unable to deal with the change, actively seek out support to help sustain you during these periods of ongoing friction.

Tempting Doctor Role
(Playing Doctor or Hey, Aren't You a Student Doctor?)

One other area requiring balance lies in your temptation to meet the family's professional expectations. During the first two years of medical school, we have very limited participation in patient care (if any). This delay can become a particularly troublesome state when family and friends start, prematurely, to expect professional expertise from you. They may ask: "What should I do for this aching knee?" "Do you think that this lump is serious?" "Is this medicine my doctor prescribed really safe?" It is flattering to be considered an expert after you've spent four months learning anatomy, but it certainly puts you in a bind to be expected to give answers that you won't have for another three or four years. So what do you do? You need to explain clearly to family members the difference between a medical student and a doctor. Give them a clear, gentle but firm message reminding them of your status and the need to delay expectations.

> Jonathan's mother had hypertension that was poorly controlled. She had a lot of questions: Was she on the correct medicine? Did she really need to take it since she felt so good? What about herbal treatments? Jonathan wisely went with her on an office visit, helping her to articulate some of her questions and reinforcing the role that her family doctor had in her care.

Children!!

Having and raising children while in medical school is a challenge. Finding the time and energy that you want to devote to them is difficult and requires careful planning. How hard will it be to manage? Is it wise (if I have a choice) to have children now? How do I handle it? Here are a few tips to keep the situation from being *too* complicated.

Start by considering a number of questions. How do I really feel about becoming/being a parent right now? It is normal to have myriad reactions: excitement, fear, joy, anger, pride, doubt, guilt, and the like. If your partner is in the picture, both of you should discuss all your respective concerns. Any hidden feelings will undoubtedly emerge right before a major exam, so get them out now. Try to develop the habit of forgiving one another for mistakes, insensitivity, and so on once aired.

Then move to the challenges of daily living ahead. What are the expectations that you and your partner have? How much of a division of labor will there be? How much time and when will you be expected to carry out parental chores? How will these responsibilities be scheduled to accommodate your exam schedules? What backup plans will you have for when your child is sick (there is no question—he or she *will* get sick). With school-age children and a working or student spouse like you, what contingency plans will you have for school holidays, school closings, and a child's illness? These questions can be answered with some forethought and with some *discussion with others who have gone through similar circumstances.*

There will be times when *guilt is unavoidable,* so expect it. You will need to (a) minimize the guilt by planning ahead and (b) accept *some* guilt as a natural event and be ready to talk about it.

Some schools provide services to help student-parents through the maze of medical school. Take advantage of these services.

Occasionally, you and your partner or spouse may need to *sit down with a counselor* to help get a better perspective on your situation. If this becomes necessary, view it as a wise move, not as a failure.

There's no "one size fits all" solution, particularly because of the way in which children's needs vary with their stages of development. The intense nurturing needed by a dependent infant is quite different from the guidance and limit setting required in dealing with a two-year-old. How children view substitute caregivers will change as the developmental levels change. It will be awfully helpful for you to get some advice from your pediatrician about the developmental needs of your children. In addition, members of the Department of Pediatrics may be glad to provide some orienting comments about where your child is coming from at a given moment. Of course, expert advice from child psychiatrists or psychologists regarding your child's emotional concerns can be enormously helpful as well.

Summary of Strategies to Balance Family and School

- Recognize the *value of family.*
- Be clear about what your role as a medical student requires. Recognize that it is necessary for you to *take on a different role in your family.*
- Be honest. *Examine all your feelings* about your life situation. With this "inventory of feelings" you can more effectively speak of the multitude of things going on in your life right now. *Accept your feelings* no matter how uncomfortable, then *work out a plan* to address your needs.

Conclusion

Ideally, the community you build in medical school will reflect your most essential parts. It can reinforce these parts of you so that you graduate a whole person, not just a doctor. If you stay connected to your community, it can support you, nurture you, and keep you growing.

NOTES

1. Drew Alexander, MD, at Southwestern Medical School.

2. Heard at the Association of American Medical Colleges Junior Faculty Development Conference, 1991.

REFERENCES

Felton, J. C. M. (1980). *The care of souls in the Black church.* New York: Martin Luther King Fellow's Press.

Grady, C. (1991). *The National Minority Mentor Recruitment Network manual* (pp. 1-16). Washington, DC: National Medical Association.

Tatum, B. D. (1997). *Why are all the Black kids sitting together in the cafeteria?* New York: Basic Books.

Wright, C. A., & Wright, S. D. (1987). The role of mentors in the career development of young professionals. *Family Relations, 36,* 204-208.

Section III
Focus on My Culture

We have considered what medical school requires and what you, the individual, will need to stay healthy academically and personally. Now let's focus on your culture. In these last pages, we take a closer look at four ethnic groups historically underrepresented in medical school: African American, Native American, Mexican American, and Puerto Rican medical students. We address your history in medicine, the contributions of your forebears, the particular challenges ahead, and secrets for your success. Finally, we consider a frank discussion of the common obstacle all minority groups face—racism—and offer practical options to manage it within this medical culture.

Focus on African American Medical Students

CARMEN WEBB, MD
STEPHANIE SMITH
MORRIS HAWKINS, JR., PHD
ANN HILL, MED

African Americans have a rich heritage in medicine. In this chapter, we will explore our history and our current status in training, including one perspective of life in a historically Black medical school. We'll examine the special challenges African American students face as well as the secrets of success used by many of our physician forebears. For the purposes of this chapter, we will use the terms *Black* and *African American* interchangeably. This includes all Black Americans of African descent, including Caribbean citizens.

History of African Americans in Medicine

Timeline (Duke University Medical Center Library, 1999; Epps, Johnson, & Vaughan,1993a, b; "Imhotep" Encyclopedia Britannica Online, 1994-2000)

As a Black student in medicine, you have a very long legacy of doctoring. For centuries, our ancestors in West Africa were called to or inherited the profession of healing. These "medicine men" or "herbalists" were trained to use herbs, minerals, and verbal/touch techniques in diagnosing and healing both physical and psychological illnesses. Families specialized in certain areas of medicine (e.g., eyes, stomach, and mouth). Their methods, although often not respected by Western medical practitioners, were developed and quite effective. Healers were counted on to be trustworthy, discerning, "upright morally, service oriented and warm" and gained the greatest respect from their community (Diop, 1987; Mbiti, 1969). The tradition of healing was not lost during slavery in America. Many plantation owners gave inadequate or no medical attention at all to slaves. Therefore, slaves combined their knowledge of African tribal medicine with Native American techniques and the "White doctor's" methods, to form their own style of medical practice (Fontenot, 1994).

Despite your rich history of physicianhood, even the consideration of your admission to formal medical training in America is hard won. As recently as the end of World War II, 26 of the 78 medical schools denied Black students admission (Shea & Fullilove, 1985). As a result, beginning in the late 1800s, eight medical schools were established to train Black students. (Although the educational opportunity was finally available, most Black students still had no choice but to travel far from home, away from community and support system.) And efforts to take our places in medicine did not stop there:

3000 B.C.
Imhotep: One of the first medicinal figures; known for his genius

1721
Onesimus: African slave with knowledge of smallpox immunization

1780
James Derham, MD: Ex-slave and first Black physician born and trained in the United States

1837
James M. Smith, MD: First African American to earn an MD

1847
David J. Peck MD: First African American to earn an MD in America

1864
Rebecca L. Crumpler, MD: First Black woman to receive an MD in the United States

1948
Edith Mae Irby, MD: First Black medical student admitted by previously segregated University of Arkansas

- **1895**—The National Medical Association (NMA) was founded. It is committed to provide "educational programs . . . outreach efforts . . . and improved public health . . . in support of Black physicians and their patients" (National Medical Association, 1999). At the time, the American Medical Association (AMA) denied Black physicians membership (Shea & Fullilove, 1985).

> "Although the practice of medicine is accorded one of the highest occupational ranks and status in America, the profession has not been able to divest itself of the subtle racism that permeates the infrastructure of our entire society." (Bullock & Houston, 1987, p. 601)

- **1948**—The University of Arkansas became the first medical school forced to accept Black students, through the efforts of the National Association for the Advancement of Colored People (NAACP) (Epps, Johnson, & Vaughan, 1993).

- **1954**—The U.S. Supreme Court desegregated public schools (Cozzens, 1998), outlawing the "separate but equal" tenet (Brown, 1958) in public education. With the introduction of affirmative action programs in the late 1960s to the mid-1970s, the number of minorities entering medical school nearly doubled.

- **1966**—The last of the still-segregated medical schools finally opened admission to minority students (Shea & Fullilove, 1985).

- **1970**—The Association of American Medical Colleges (AAMC) made a commitment to try to equate the number of entering minority students in medical school to a comparable percentage of the total population (AAMC Task Force, 1970). This required that entering classes contain approximately 12% Black students (Shea & Fullilove, 1985).

- **1978**—Allen Bakke, a White applicant, stated that his denial of admission to medical school was a violation of the Fourteenth Amendment. Thereafter, the Supreme Court ruled that "quotas were [not] necessary to achieve diversity" (Motley, 1979). As a result, the numbers of Black Americans entering medical school remained at approximately 9% of all entrants until 1990.

- **1991**—The AAMC launched Project 3000 by 2000 (AAMC, 1996). The goal is "to increase the number of underrepresented minority (URM) students entering the nation's 125 medical schools each year to 3,000 by the year 2000" (p. 1).

Although we've seen great change in opportunities for medical education since 1895, the tide again has begun to turn:

- **1996**—Californians voted to ban affirmative action (Proposition 209) (Academic Affairs Human Resources, 1998).

- **1997**—The Supreme Court supported the ruling in *Hopwood v. Texas* (1994), leading to denying consideration of race and ethnicity in higher education admissions in Texas, Louisiana, and Mississippi.

These decisions have decreased the number of Black entrants to medical school, although the total number of entrants across all races has increased (AAMC, 1999).

Current Status

Even as we are repeatedly challenged to maintain the tremendous strides we've gained thus far, African American physicians continue to achieve excellence in a variety of settings. Mae C. Jemison, MD, a 1981 graduate of the Cornell University School of Medicine, became the first Black female astronaut in NASA history in August 1988. Ben Carson, MD, a 1987 graduate of the University of Michigan Medical school became the first pediatric neurosurgeon of any race to successfully separate Siamese twins joined at the back of the head (Carson & Murphey, 1990). Other greats of this decade include pediatric endocrinologist Joycelyn Elders, MD, a 1960 graduate of Arkansas Medical School, who became the first African American Surgeon General in 1993. In 1997, Paula Mahone, MD, and Karen Drake, MD, were the first physicians to deliver living septuplets. Clearly, the contributions by Black physicians are essential. However, at the time of this writing, the percentage of Black students in medical schools is still far below the 12.6% of Blacks in the total U.S. population (AAMC, 1999; Division of Community and Minority Programs, 1998, p. 113).

Historically Black medical schools (HBMSs) have remained invested in increasing this percentage. Of the original eight HBMSs, two remain: Howard University College of Medicine, founded in 1867, and Meharry Medical College, founded in 1876. Two schools were added in the latter half of the 20th century to train the growing numbers of Black applicants: Charles R. Drew University of Medicine and Science (1966) and Morehouse College of Medicine (1978). If you are one of the many African Americans who choose an HBMS, what might you expect?

Perspective: Life in a Historically Black Medical School

Life in an HBMS offers a unique experience. Of course, students in any medical school share similarities: You have been accepted into a medical education curriculum. You must pay tuition and fees (although your sources of revenue may vary), take required and elective courses, and pass board and licensure examinations. However, because African Americans constitute the majority in an HBMS, a greater number of students than in majority schools may share your background, both economically and socially. You have similar tastes in style of dress and gastronomical pleasures. You may even have similar stress levels and problem-solving skills. The questions about "am I being treated differently from my peers because I am Black?" no longer apply.

> "At our school, we experience a socialization into a new culture—'The Family of Howard Doctors.'"

Relationships. The camaraderie at an HBMS is extremely important. Students usually need to pool and share resources. You find yourself a roommate or two. You share transportation (especially if you don't own a car), so you leave and return home at the same time many days. Even though you are in a competitive environment, you tend to share notes, references, old examinations, and often use a study group.

An HBMS usually extends itself to minorities from Third World countries. Therefore, the student body includes African Americans, Blacks from island and African nations, Hispanics, Pacific Islanders, Asians, Native Americans, and European Americans. Students tend to want to share their cultures and cultural habits. You learn to eat different foods at meals (sometimes), you experience the uses and wearing of different apparel, and you even may learn a different dance step or two. Non-Black students are readily integrated into the educational environment and hence may not feel the degree of isolation and segregation that Black students face at majority institutions.

Interestingly enough, all types of employees seem to get along at an HBMS. Domestic and security staff, audiovisual and building maintenance, office and administrative secretaries, all seem to get close to one student or another. They become a part of the extended support system. Each group learns to respect the other, and members of the group feel as if they are part of a unit, all trying to accomplish the same thing.

Academics. Don't think for a minute that the HBMS is more social than serious. Certainly, the socialization process is a bit easier to navigate, but remember, all schools are held to the same curricular standards. An HBMS takes these standards *very* seriously and works very hard to ensure that you meet them. You are assigned a sophomore student adviser who gives you a heads up on how to make it through the first year and into the second year success-

You are also assigned a faculty adviser. Most individual faculty members are very accessible. An HBMS is heavily dependent on faculty and medical officers for teaching and training, primarily because they have smaller numbers of clinical and volunteer faculty. Thus, students interact very closely with professors, receiving firsthand advice, academic help, and career counseling. The faculty at an HBMS is quite diverse; usually 30% or more are Caucasian or international. This diversity makes it much easier to provide role models for all ethnic groups. Also, you can find a medical education office that offers a comprehensive set of support services to meet the needs of all students, whether or not they are struggling. (Unlike majority schools, there is no such position at an HBMS as an assistant dean for minority affairs.) All administrators are thus focused on educational goals that address all students.

Conclusion. Historically Black medical schools provide a solid foundation in medicine as well as a uniquely supportive socialization. They produce excellent physicians.

Special Challenges

You will face a number of challenges as an African American medical student.

"I was so tired during exam week. After one test, a Caucasian physician that I was shadowing sat me down in his office and proceeded to inform me that it would be difficult especially as a Black female to enter his area of medicine. He then asked, "So what do you want to go into?" I said nothing because I was not thinking about the implications of his words. I just wanted to go home and take a nap. Later, when speaking to my mentor, I realized how derogatory that interaction was. I had not defended myself because I was too tired. Because of my silence, he probably thought that I was OK with what he had said and he would not feel bad about saying it to someone else."

Racism

Racism is common in medical culture (Schulman et al., 1999; Weiss, 1999), just as it is in other areas of society (see Chapter 12). Even if you have learned to cope with racial injustices in the past, you will likely find it more difficult to do so while trying to navigate the medical school curriculum. The literature suggests that Black students report mistreatment to a greater degree than do majority students (Richardson, Becker, Frank, & Sokol, 1997). In the context of medical culture, it may be particularly tricky to determine whether you are being mistreated because you are Black or because you are a student (low in the hierarchy). Or you may discover that you stop coping effectively because you simply stop caring about racism (Slavin, Ranier, McCreary, & Gowda, 1991).

Identity Development

During the clinical years, you will be formulating your identity as a Black physician. The disproportionately small number of Black physician role models, as well as the lack of support from the majority culture, might challenge this development, especially if you attend a majority school (Bonnett & Douglas, 1983; Nager & Saadatmand, 1991; Strayhorn, 1981). Sometimes, you may struggle with the "Eurocentric" view (achievement in individual pursuits) versus the "Afrocentric" view (meeting the needs of the group) (Post & Weddington, 1997). You may even question your choice of career, wondering if those in your ethnic group belong in medicine.

> It is a particular sensation, this double-consciousness, one ever feels his two-ness—an American, a Negro; two souls, two unreconciled strivings, two warring ideals in one dark body, whose dogged strength alone keeps it from being torn asunder. (Du Bois, 1903, p. 5)

On the other hand, your values might be more closely aligned with mainstream views, especially in terms of time and activity (Shervington, Bland, & Myers, 1996). Perhaps you hoped that once you became a professional, you would be granted all the privileges of upper-middle-class society. "Yet all Black Americans, regardless of income or professional achievements, are occasionally reminded that because of race there are things in society that wealth cannot provide" (Carter, 1992, p. 32). This dilemma adds extra stress to the already stressful academic environment and could be one of the factors that leads to diminished academic performance in school (Rico & Stagnaro-Green, 1997).

Responsibility: "You Are Black. You Should Give Back"

Now that you are in medical school, you have likely been encouraged to continue to follow your dreams. On the other hand, you may also have been told that those Black physicians who are in the position to help their community and the underserved, should do so (Carter, 1992). Others' expectations of you might impose substantial pressure to succeed and to serve—or else let the entire Black community down (see Chapter 4).

Playtime

When you finally put down the books and take the time to play, you may find yourself at a loss. If you find it most relaxing to kick back with other Blacks but attend a school with few African Americans, you may long for that outlet. As one student commented, "I tried the medical school parties, but they centered around drinking or standing around talking. My idea of a good party is lots of music and dancing." If you are in an HBMS, there may be many opportunities for socializing in the university around you. Your struggle will be to find a good balance between school and work.

> "I was feeling so grungy and tired after my surgery rotation. My (Caucasian) upper year suggested she'd always felt better if she got her hair done. I didn't have the energy to tell her that for me it meant a half-hour drive across town to find a Black hairstylist and then a few hours in the chair. She didn't understand that I just couldn't go to a local place and be out in half an hour."

Resources

The products and people that Blacks need to maintain their hair, the availability of particular foods, and the difficulty they may have in finding a church of their choosing are all challenges that may not be obvious to the majority community.

Romantic Relationships

Simply finding a partner in medical school may be difficult. If you are looking for someone with whom you are compatible and who is also Black, you may find yourself combing the community for someone who is available but not threatened by your professional status or your time limitations. Dating another medical student (if people to choose from are present) can be convenient, but it leaves your relationship open to scrutiny and, at times, the involvement of the larger medical school community. If you are interested in someone outside your race, your options may be greater, but you must be ready for sometimes critical responses by Blacks and non-Blacks alike. Once in a relationship, if you are African American with an African American partner, your new identity/role as a professional may be muddied by Dumas's

(1979) "hydraulic system of male/female relationships. . . . Black males can rise only to the degree that Black women are held down" (p. 204). If the Black woman attempts to progress, she may be labeled as the "strong, uppidy, castrating Black woman" (Dumas, 1979). Alternatively, the successful, focused Black man may be accused of disregarding his partner. Roles of men and women in African American and Caribbean and African traditions can be quite different, and couples expecting sameness based on skin color are surprised, disappointed, or just confused. Certainly, relationships do survive medical school but usually only with a great deal of foresight, effort, and commitment.

Finances

The financial burden of Blacks in medical school is often greater than for White students (Rico & Stagnaro-Green, 1997). There are still relatively few Black families who have enjoyed many generations of financial security; therefore, there are fewer families who are financially stable enough to offer monetary help. Even those who have resources may be limited because they must also assist others in the family. Furthermore, if your family is part of the Black middle class, you may not be eligible for financial aid based solely on need. If your family is unable to assist you financially (or is not able to provide enough), you will likely choose to work. This, of course, can interfere considerably with study and personal time.

Secrets of Success:
Advice From Fifty Black Physicians

Despite the challenges, many Black physicians have made it. Your graduation from medical school will in itself also be a success story. One of this chapter's authors (Smith) conducted structured telephone interviews with 50 Black physicians across the country to learn how they managed personal and/or academic obstacles during medical school. Interestingly, the methods that these physicians identified are the same ones that have contributed to success for Blacks throughout history.

Know Your Legacy

African history emphasizes the wisdom of elders who have traveled the same path and willingly share their knowledge of pitfalls (Malidoma, 1988;

Raboteau, 1978). Because trying to handle medical school without guidance is close to impossible, seek out individuals who can guide you along the way. Make it your business to pay attention to accomplishments of other Black physicians (even if these contributions are not publicly celebrated). Have friends and family send you stories and news of African American physicians' accomplishments. You may be surprised at how motivating this can be. The achievements of others can help you to set new goals for yourself and to look beyond that next exam.

Draw Strength From the Community

Ask for help. The model of care in African tradition is that one can, if necessary, count on resources in the family/tribe/clan/town for assistance. Historically, all members of the community had duties and responsibilities to one another (Felton, 1980; Mbiti, 1969, 1991). Similarly, almost to a person, the physicians surveyed believed it crucial to seek help. Their advice? Don't wait until you are in emotional or academic trouble to admit that you need others; look for it from the beginning. Do not allow yourself to become isolated because you don't do the legwork required to find good resources.

Seriously consider a study group, even if you've never used one before. Choose people of all races who are high achievers. Observe their approaches to study, and know your own strengths and weaknesses (Massey, 1992).

You may find the Student National Medical Association (SNMA) the main path to your service, social, and networking options. The oldest and largest student organization focused on the concerns of medical students of color, it offers many minority students support and comradeship. Its programs are designed to meet the health needs of the underrepresented community and to promote culturally sensitive mediation and services (SNMA, 1999).

Remember to draw from the *whole* community. That is, do not overlook the advice and knowledge of nonphysicians. Those nurses, ward clerks, security guards, and cafeteria and maintenance workers who have been involved with the institution for years also have secrets of success that can help you. These are the individuals to whom you turn when you need to gain access to a room or when you are unsure of what happened to your lab results. Sometimes they are the ones who will listen to you vent your frustrations.

Draw on Spiritual Strength

In African culture, the spiritual is as important as the physical (Felton, 1980; Mbiti, 1991). During slavery, this orientation continued with input from

White America. Today, spiritual growth is reported as central to the success of many African Americans (Fraser, 1998; Nivins, 1998). A survey of 15 Black residents revealed that as medical students, they frequently coped with difficulty on the wards by "praying" or "finding new faith" (Shields & Webb, 1993).

You may, as do some medical students, be tempted to forego your religious and spiritual heritage, whatever it is, because you assume that that is what medical culture requires. On the contrary, many African American physicians in Smith's research felt that spirituality had been a major source of their strength. Said one, "You have so many new and tremendous challenges in medical school, you would be foolish to give up any resource that you have now."

Be in Control of Your Response to Racism

Through strategically planned efforts, Black Americans have made tremendous strides against racism (the Underground Railroad, the Civil Rights Movement) in our society (Robinson, 1997). You also need to have controlled responses to the racism that you experience in medical culture (see Chapter 12). Your ability to manage your response will help you to maximize your power over seemingly uncontrollable circumstances. For example, although you are grieving the absence (because of racism) of a professor's high regard, use the experience to remind you to fight, not to eventually gain someone's respect—you have very limited control over that—but for excellence in medical knowledge and skill. Then no matter how you are regarded, you will have the expertise to be an outstanding physician. Try to prevent the personal thoughts and opinions of others from clouding your focus. By minimizing the negative thoughts provoked by a perpetrator of racism, you will grow stronger with each encounter. This "racial inoculation," similar to the medical concept of inoculation, allows you to build a strong resistance against attacks and thus learn to avoid victimization (Finley & Pernell-Arnold, 1997).

Maintain Who You Are and Where You Are Going

Even in the midst of slavery, Blacks strove to maintain personal identity. By preserving their culture, they could thereby "preserve some personal autonomy . . . and resist infantilization, total identification" with slave owners (Blassingame, 1972). Years later, with the recurring setbacks and with the constant assaults on personal dignity and on life itself, the civil rights effort certainly might have been derailed. However, those fighting ultimately won because they stayed focused on their goals (Carson, Garrow, Gill, Harding, & Hine, 1991).

Establish from the beginning exactly who you are and why you are valuable to the world. Take time to examine the ethnic, racial, social, physical, psychological, and spiritual parts of yourself that you wish to be intact by the time you graduate. Make it your business to do those things you need to do to maintain them. By cherishing your strengths in other areas of your life (Nivins, 1998), you can formulate the contributions you plan to make in the future. The firmer these plans are, the less likely you are to be sidetracked by obstacles or to let others' opinions define your goals for you (keeping your eyes on the prize) (Carson et al., 1991). Then write a phrase, say a word, draw a picture—anything that reminds you of your importance and of your goals. Post these reminders everywhere (on your notebooks, in your bathroom, in your locker) so that you can refer to them often during the challenges of medical study.

Adapt Quickly

Throughout history, Black Americans have learned and taught their offspring how to adapt and survive in bondage, segregation, discrimination, and in the White middle-class structure (Blassingame, 1972). During slavery, children learned to adopt the mask of deferential speech and actions with their owners. Even now, many African Americans learn two modes of speech to "make it" in the majority society and to be trusted in the Black community. Adaptability further involves finding resources when you have limited options—"making a way out of no way" as Blacks have done for centuries (Hale, 1982). Families with flexibility and creativity are those that survive (Pinderhughes, 1982).

Similarly, your ability to adapt quickly to medical culture, and to each of the specialty subcultures on the wards, will aid greatly in your success. It may be tempting to defy all the rules you disapprove (see Chapters 1 and 3). Don't. Assess quickly the dictums of the new environment (ask upper years; observe closely) and adjust to those that are critical to your academic survival. Assess any academic areas that you need to strengthen and fortify. You do not have time to hold on to your pride, if you really need to change your study patterns (Bullock & Houston, 1987; Reitzes & Elkhanialy, 1976), play less or get a tutor. *Your primary objective is to learn the material and to earn your M.D. degree.* Therefore, oppose the cultural dictums only if you have counted the cost and are willing to accept the consequences. Still, even slaves were not unconditionally submissive, and some were willing to die to protect one another (Blassingame, 1972). Successful adaptation does not mean giving up your own culture. Make a point to express your beliefs and values when away from school. (Dress the way you prefer; speak the way you choose.) You have a legacy of adaptation. It will serve you well.

Get Organized and "Just Do It"

Many African American physicians interviewed related their success to a phrase that exasperated parents have said to their children for years: "Just do it." When you have made adjustments to your attitude, tried to draw on strength from within, and worked to get help from without, yet medical school still feels endless, sometimes the only thing left is to "just do it." If this is the case, you'll need to put emotional distance between yourself and your behavior. This may allow you to separate your feelings about the social situation from your work and may be enough to get you through (Bullock & Houston, 1987).

The ability to *just do it* requires organization. Many physicians in the survey pointed out that they found no time in medical school for sloppy habits. Similarly, one focus group of students from an HBMS emphasized that a large part of organization was "getting your life in order." Work out that family relationship, get rid of that useless boyfriend or girlfriend, get over that poor self-concept, because once you matriculate, you don't have time to put significant work into fixing these areas.

What African Americans Offer the World of Medicine

Black physicians have a wealth of achievements in medicine. Some are well-known: Samuel Lee Kountz, Jr., MD; Louis Sullivan, MD; and Charles Richard Drew, MD Others are less widely promoted. Yet their care of patients, research contributions, and administrative skills are all gifts to the world of medicine.

Some studies report that physicians are most comfortable with patients whom they perceive as similar to themselves and are uncomfortable with patients whom they perceive as different (Gregory, Wells, & Leake, 1987). On the other hand, many Black physicians have had to negotiate both Black and White cultures and may offer medicine a physician who is comfortable with a wider range of patient populations. Furthermore, medical school culture emphasizes individualism, autonomy, reality, and mastery. By contrast, the African American cultural heritage is rich with ingenuity, adaptability, family, spirituality, and sharing. The literature reports that these qualities in a physician are central to patient satisfaction (Bailey, 1987). Finally, non-minority students and physicians can draw from our legacy of strength in the midst of difficult circumstances. The same secrets of success mentioned earlier that Black Americans have used for centuries can be helpful to non-Black students and physicians today.

A non-African American student, who had been feeling discouraged and frustrated with medical school, came in one day with renewed motivation. When questioned, she reported excitedly how inspired she was after finishing the book *Gifted Hands* by Benjamin Carson, M.D. She was encouraged by seeing that he had overcome so many challenges and felt she could now do the same.

Conclusion

As an African American medical student, you can make a very definite contribution to the world of medicine. Your legacy of excellent Black physicians is available for example and inspiration. Their journey required strength and persistence, and their success is testimony that it can be done. The wisdom of these men and women is waiting for you as you take your place in medicine.

REFERENCES

Academic Affairs Human Resources, University of California. (1998). *Implementation of Proposition 209: How it impacts UC's employment practices.* University of California, Office of the President. http://www.ucop.edu/humres/policies/sp-2.html
Association of American Medical Colleges & Division of Community and Minority Programs (1996, April). *Project 3000 by 2000.* Washington, DC: Author. http://www.aamc.org/meded/minority/3x2/fouryear.htm#introduction
Association of American Medical Colleges. (1999). *New entrants by gender and race/ethnicity* [table]. http://www.aamc.org/stuapps/facts/famg7.htm

Association of American Medical Colleges Task Force. (1970). *Report of the Association of American Medical Colleges Task Force to the Inter-Association Committee on Expanding Educational Opportunities in Medicine for Blacks and Other Minority Students.* Washington, DC: AAMC.

Bailey, E. J. (1987). Sociocultural factors and health care-seeking behavior among Black Americans. *Journal of the National Medical Association, 79*(4), 389-392.

Blassingame, J. (1972). *The slave community.* New York: Oxford University Press.

Bonnett, A. W., & Douglas, F. L. (1983, Summer). Black medical students in White medical schools. *Social Policy,* pp. 23-26.

Brown, J. H. B. (1958). Majority opinion in *Plessy v. Ferguson.* In B. M. Ziegler (Ed.), *Desegregation and the Supreme Court* (pp. 50-51). Boston: D. C. Heath.

Bullock, S. C., & Houston, E. (1987). Perceptions of racism by Black medical students attending White medical schools. *Journal of the National Medical Association, 79*(6), 601-608.

Carson, C., Garrow, D. J., Gill, G., Harding, V., & Hine, D. C. (1991). *The eyes on the prize civil rights reader.* New York: Penguin.

Carson, B., & Murphey, C. (1990). *Gifted hands: The Ben Carson story.* Grand Rapids, MI: Zondervan.

Carter, J. H. (1992). Black health professional families: Assessment of strengths and stability. *Journal of the National Medical Association, 84*(1), 31-35.

Cozzens, L. (1998). *Brown v. Board of Education.* http://www.fledge.watson.org/~lisa/blackhistory/early-civilrights/brown.html

Diop, C. A. (1987). *Pre-Colonial Black Africa.* Brooklyn, NY: Lawrence Hill.

Division of Community and Minority Programs. (1998). *Minority students in medical education: Facts and figures* (Vol. XI). Washington, DC: Association of American Medical Colleges.

Du Bois, W. E. B. (1903). *Souls of Black folk.* Chicago: McClurg.

Duke University Center Medical Center Library. (1999). *Chronology of achievements of African Americans in medicine.* www.mc.duke.edu/mclibrary/hot/bhmtime.html

Dumas, R. (1979). The dilemma of the gifted woman. *Journal of Personality and Social Systems, 2*(1), 203-214.

Epps, C. H., Johnson, D. G., & Vaughan, A. L. (1993). Black medical pioneers: Part 1. African-American "firsts" in academic and organized medicine. *Journal of the National Medical Association, 85*(8), 629-644.

Epps, C. H., Johnson, D. G., & Vaughan, A. L. (1993). Black medical pioneers, Part 2: African-American "firsts" in academic and organized medicine. *Journal of the National Medical Association, 85*(9), 703-720.

Felton, J. C. M. (1980). *The care of souls in the Black church.* New York: Martin Luther King Fellow's Press.

Finley, L., & Pernell-Arnold, A. (1997, August). *Multicultural research and training institute.* Paper presented at the annual meeting of the American Psychological Association, Chicago.

Fontenot, W. L. (1994). *Secret doctors: Ethnomedicine of African Americans.* Westport, CT: Bergin & Garvey.

Fraser, G. C. (1998). *Race for success: The ten best business opportunities for Blacks in America.* New York: William Morrow.

Gregory, K., Wells, K., & Leake, B. (1987). Medical students' expectations for encounters with minority and nonminority patients. *Journal of the National Medical Association, 79*(4), 403-408.

Hale, J. E. (1982). *Black children: Their roots, culture and learning styles.* Baltimore: Johns Hopkins University Press.

Hopwood v. Texas (861 F. Supp. 551 W.D. Tex. 1994).

"Imhotep" Encyclopedia Britannica Online. (copyright 1994-2000). http://search.eb.com/bol.topic?eu=43134&setn=1 (accessed 23 May 2000).

Malidoma, P. S. (1998). *The healing wisdom of Africa.* New York: Jeremy P. Tarcher/Putnam.

Massey, W. E. (1992). Minorities in science two generations of struggle. *Science, 258,* 1176-1218.

Mbiti, J. S. (1969). *African religions and philosophy.* Portsmouth, NH: Heinemann.

Mbiti, J. S. (1991). *Introduction to African religion.* London: Heinemann.

Motley, C. (1979). From Brown to Bakke: The long road to equality. *Harvard Civil Rights—Civil Liberties Law Review, 14,* 315-327.

Nager, N., & Saadatmand, F. (1991). The status of medical education for Black Americans. *Journal of National Medical Association, 83,* 787-792.

Nivins, B. (1998). *Success strategies for African Americans.* New York: Plume.

Pinderhughes, E. B. (1982). Family functioning of Afro-Americans. *Social Work, 27*(1), 83-90.

Post, D., & Weddington, W. (1997). The impact of culture on physician stress and coping. *Journal of the National Medical Association, 89*(9), 585-590.

Raboteau, A. (1978). *Slave religion.* Oxford, UK: Oxford University Press.

Reitzes, D., & Elkhanialy, H. (1976). Black students in medical schools. *Journal of Medical Education, 51*(12), 1001-1005.

Richardson, D. A., Becker, M., Frank, R. R., & Sokol, R. J. (1997). Assessing medical studeⱡits' perceptions of mistreatment in their second and third years. *Academic Medicine, 72*(8), 728-730.

Rico, M., & Stagnaro-Green, A. (1997). Debt and career choices of underrepresented minorities. *Academic Medicine, 72*(8), 657-659.

Robinson, C. J. (1997). *Black movements in America.* New York: Routledge.

Schulman, K., Berlin, J., Harless, W., Kerner, J., Sistrunk, S., Gersh, B., Dube, R., Taleghani, C., Burke, J., Williams, S., Eisenberg, J., & Escarce, J. (1999). The effect of race and sex on physicians' recommendations for cardiac catheterization. *New England Journal of Medicine, 340*(8), 618-626.

Shea, S., & Fullilove, M. T. (1985). Entry of Black and other minority students into U.S. medical schools. *New England Journal of Medicine, 313*(15), 933-940.

Shervington, D. O., Bland, I. J., & Myers, A. (1996). Ethnicity, gender identity, stress, and coping among female African-American medical students. *Journal of the American Medical Women's Association, 51*(4), 153-154.

Shields, P., & Webb, C. (1993). [Ways of Coping Scale administered to residents]. Unpublished raw data.

Slavin, L. A. R., Ranier, K. L. McCreary, M. L. Gowda, K. K. (1991). Toward a multicultural model of the stress process. *Journal of Counseling and Development, 70,* 156-163.

Strayhorn, G. (1980). Social supports, perceived stress, and health: The Black experience in medical school—A preliminary study. *Journal of the National Medical Association, 72*(9), 869-881.

Student National Medical Association. (1999). http://www.snma.org

Weiss, J. (1999, June 1). Doctors grapple with biases. *Dallas Morning News,* pp. 1A and 7A.

Focus on
Native American
Medical Students

LORI ARVISO ALVORD, MD

In the largest sense, the definition of *Native American* is an individual who is a member of a tribe of people indigenous to the Americas. For the purposes of this chapter, we are referring only to tribes living in the United States. Each tribe determines its own tribal membership requirements. Most require a specific blood quantum or require that parents or grandparents be enrolled tribal members.

History of Native Americans
in Medicine

The First Native American Physicians

Historical data regarding the training of physicians who were Native American are hard to find prior to 1974, when the Association of American Medical Colleges (AAMC) began collecting careful data about underrepresented

156

minorities in medical school. However, certain individual Native American physicians are well recognized because they are the first members of their tribes to become physicians. One of the earliest physicians on record is Charles Eastman, the first Lakota physician. He received his M.D. degree from Boston University in 1890 (Badt, 1995). Other examples include Lorette Helle, credited as the first Native Alaskan physician, who received her M.D. in 1958 (Durrett, 1997, p. 74), and Taylor McKenzie, the first Navajo physician, who received his degree in 1958 (Iverson, 1981).

Who Is a Native American?

The AAMC keeps records of the numbers of Native American students accepted into medical school and keeps other important information relating to the historical and current status of Native American students. A word of caution regarding the interpretation of this data is necessary, however. The AAMC asks Native Americans to "self-identify" on the admissions application for medical school. No other verification of Native American identity is required. Problems arise in trying to determine which students should be considered Native American. It is not uncommon for individuals to claim Native American heritage even though they may have minimal blood quantum and no cultural or community association with Native groups. Admissions committees at some schools believe that the self-identification process tends to skew the data on numbers of Native American students and leads to an artificially inflated pool of students. (I have served on admissions committees at Dartmouth Medical School and Stanford Medical School and have served as a consultant to the undergraduate admissions committee at Dartmouth College. At each institution, this situation has arisen, and has served as a topic for much discussion and debate.) The ethical questions surrounding this problem are complicated and will not be addressed in depth here. It is clear, however, that Native American tribes and communities would prefer that medical schools train individuals who have maintained a relationship with their respective tribes or who have some understanding of the culture with which they self-identify. Admissions committees face the dilemma of how to determine which applicants are merely claiming to be Native Americans to improve their chances of admission. The undergraduate admissions committee at Dartmouth College has developed a questionnaire for students who claim to be Native American to help them determine the strength of a student's Native American background. (This questionnaire is included at the end of this chapter.)

Current Status

How Many Native American Students
Are Accepted to Medical School?

According to the AAMC (1996) in 1974, 64 Native Americans were accepted into medical schools in the United States (of a total of 15,066 acceptances.) This number has steadily risen over the years, and in 1996, 134 Native American students were accepted into medical schools (of a total of 17,385). This increase corresponds to an increase in the number of applications: In 1974, 134 Native American students applied, compared with 1996, when 323 students applied. Acceptance rates have declined slightly as a percentage over the years: In 1974, 47% of the Native American applicant pool was accepted, compared with 41% in 1996. (The acceptance rate peaked to a high of 61% in 1989 but has dropped steadily since then. The acceptance rate for White students rose during that time as well, to 61%.) The percentage of acceptance rates is higher for Native Americans than the rates for White students: In 1974, 34% of White students were accepted, and in 1996, 38% of White students were accepted.

Special Challenges

Inadequate Academic Preparation
for Medical School

Many Native American students come from disadvantaged backgrounds. A number of students come from low-income communities with high schools that lack adequate funding and staffing, leading to inadequate preparation for students when they reach college. Therefore, students may spend much of college "catching up," and this period may extend into medical school. Many of you are the first members of your families to obtain a college degree or to enter postgraduate training. If this is true for you, you will probably need to spend more time studying than other medical students, to achieve satisfactory grades. Some of you will be stunned to find that an "adequate" amount of studying in medical school represents far more time than you spent studying as undergraduates. Because academic abilities are frequently linked with your self-confidence, if you are struggling academically, you may have problems with low morale as well. This sometimes causes students to withdraw from medical school. For this reason, you should seek assistance early if you are having academic trouble rather than waiting to see if you sink or swim. In general, if you are a student who is now in medical school, you were accepted based on a prior academic record that indicates that you have a good chance of completing medical school successfully. You may need to be reminded that you have "got what it takes." If you are in the process of choosing a medical school and you think this may be a problem, you should consider choosing a school that has resources available to help you improve your learning and study skills (such as tutorial assistance, learning skills centers, etc.)

Social Adjustment Problems

When you begin medical school, you may develop feelings of isolation and loneliness. Although this happens most acutely as undergraduates (unless you happen to attend a college close to home), the problem may continue in medical school. It is one of the most common reasons for students to have academic difficulty or to withdraw from school. This issue is particularly difficult for Native Americans for at least four reasons:

Lack of Other Native Students. The number of Native Americans in medical schools are so few that often there may be only one in a class. Even if there are more, other Native students will likely come from other tribes so that you may have little in common with the other students. The AAMC reports that Native American students represented less than 1% of the medical student body in 1996.

Difference in Communication. Many Native people are naturally reticent. This is part of our cultural belief system in which silence is valued as much as speech, the weight of each word carries significant meaning, and an easy dialogue is encountered only between individuals who know one another well. You may find that non-Natives interpret this communication difference as aloofness or hostility. In fact, communication styles can sometimes be so radically different that you may find the behavior of your fellow students and faculty members offensive when they ask questions that you may consider too personal or none of their business. Native Americans often treat personal information much like personal property; it may be given as a "gift," but it should not be requested. Even such seemingly innocuous questions as, "So what did you do last Saturday night?" or "That sure was a nice girl you were with the other day" may be considered invasions of privacy unless a friendship is already well established (the implication being that the person making the statement would like to know more about the student's personal life).

Belonging to a Tribe. Many of you come from communities where tribal life is considered as important as individual life and where individuals are part of a larger "living organism"—the tribe. Therefore, when you leave your tribe, you may develop an acute sense of detachment. Separated from your tribe, you may have trouble thriving. By contrast, in the Western world, you will find that a higher value is placed on independence and autonomy, and over the past 50 years, families have become very mobile. This mobility leads some individuals to have little sense of belonging to a community, and most have no comprehension or appreciation of what it means to belong to a tribe. Tribal connections can be very hard for the Western world to comprehend or appreciate, but they are a very real part of many cultures.

A Spiritual Relationship With the Land. Many Native American tribes have very close ties to the land—the places that they come from. The deep relationship with land and the rest of the environment often has a spiritual component. Consequently, it can be as difficult for students to be away from the land as it is to be away from their families (Bazhonoodah, 1978). Additionally, students from wide open spaces like the plains or the deserts of the Southwest may have a very difficult time living in areas where the horizon is obscured by buildings, trees, mountains, or other objects. They frequently describe a kind of claustrophobia that results from being away from their usual surroundings. It is likely that the reverse is also true—that students from mountainous areas may be uncomfortable in areas where the horizon stretches for many miles.

Differences in Dress or Appearance

Another problem that you may face results from differences in dress or appearance. The most striking example is the custom of men who wear their hair long. Although this has become much more acceptable in mainstream society, in Native culture, the men of some tribes have kept their hair long as a result of traditional cultural practices. Some members of American society (often those viewed as being more "radical" than the mainstream) have chosen to wear their hair long as a sign of rebellion against society, or as a fashion statement. Native people do this as part of a larger system of cultural beliefs, some of which have spiritual elements as well. You might encounter professors leading small-group sessions or attending professors while on clinical rotations in hospitals who may have negative opinions about males with long hair.

Differences in Values

As you enter the higher educational environment, you may find yourself in situations that challenge your core values. In many Native cultures, it is impolite to be overtly competitive, and students will often "hide" their accomplishments or scholastic capabilities to avoid seeming arrogant or proud or to avoid calling attention to themselves. Many will not raise their hands to answer questions even when they know the answer. This is especially true when doing so might make another student look bad or have his or her feelings hurt as a result of the actions of the first student (Durmont, 1972; Erickson & Mohatt, 1982; Ness, 1981). Some examples of research that support these observations follow. Wax (1971) noted that

> Indian peoples hesitate to engage in an individual performance before the public gaze, especially where they sense competitive assessment against their peers. Indian children do not wish to be exposed as inadequate before their peers, and equally do not wish to demonstrate by their individual superiority the inferiority of their peers. On the other hand, when performance is socially defined as benefiting the peer society, Indians become excellent competitors (as witnessed by their success in team athletics). (p. 85)

Havighurst (1970) found that "Indian children may not parade their knowledge before others or try to appear better than their peers" (p. 109). Many Native people place very little emphasis on personal gain and will deemphasize self-advancement in favor of family and community advancement. In some tribes, a person who becomes too wealthy or prominent risks being accused of witchcraft or of benefiting at the expense of others (Kluckhohn, 1967; Simmons, 1974). Therefore, students may have ambivalent feelings about publicizing their educational achievements as well. In fact, some Native American professionals have returned to their homes only to be ostracized by their family and peers. (This phenomenon does not happen to only Native Americans. Other individuals who come from similar communities will often find themselves ostracized or ridiculed, as people "back home" believe that "you think you're better than we are," etc.) In fact, some Native American students have so much ambivalence about this that they have put off or delayed getting their professional degrees.

Differences in Learning and Communication Styles and in Cultural Taboos

If you come from certain tribes, you may have been taught different norms of social conduct when it comes to interacting with others, and this may interfere with your learning environment. Prolonged eye contact is often considered rude, as is approaching another person too closely (the "private space" around Native Americans is often a larger circle than most Americans are used to). You may appear to be remote, or people might think you are avoiding them. Some cultures interpret eye contact as "honest communication"; the avoidance of eye contact can be interpreted as a dishonest demeanor or that Native people are trying to hide something.

Many Native students are raised with communication, learning, and interaction methods that differ radically from methods frequently used by the Western world. For example, in traditional communities, elders provide teachings about life, and those who are learning listen quietly without interruption as a mark of respect. It is considered rude to ask preliminary questions or interrupt, because it is generally felt that the teachers will answer most questions eventually and at the correct time (Biondel, 1980).

You may find that medical school faculty members will often view students from such backgrounds as passive, too quiet, disinterested, noninteractive, and so on. Native children are frequently taught to watch and observe for longer periods of time, and because of this difference, you may be labeled as a student who "holds back" or who is reluctant to get involved with group learning, when you merely have a different style of learning. Again, research supports these learning differences. Wax observed that "Indians tend to ridicule the person who performs clumsily. An individual should not attempt an action unless he knows how to do it, and if he does not know, then he should watch until he has understood. In European and American culture generally, the opposite attitude is usually the case, we 'give a man credit for trying' and we feel that the way to learn is to attempt to do so" (Wax & Wax, 1964, pp. 95-96). You may find yourself wondering why you are reluctant to risk failure in front of others. Appleton (1983) observed that Yaqui children are encouraged to learn by watching and modeling: "learning the correct way to do a task by watching it being performed repeatedly by others is highly reinforced" (p. 173). Therefore, it should not surprise you if you prefer to see something done many times before trying it yourself. Education researchers have documented that Native American children from the Southwestern tribes have a highly visual approach to learning (John, 1972).

Phileon and Galloway (1969) reported that children displayed remarkable ability in visual discrimination. By imitating the behaviors of others, very young children (4 yr. and 5 yr.) were able to perform complicated sets of actions without verbal directions. Kleinfield (1973) described the extraordinary accuracy of Eskimos in memory of visual information. Therefore, you might have difficulty adapting to situations where you are expected to "learn as you go." This is the way that medical schools teach procedures, and it is also a technique used for teaching students how to present data about patients on rounds in the clinical years. On the other hand, you may find you have exceptional abilities in visual learning such as anatomy, surgery, or any area where concepts are easily visualized (biochemistry, genetics, etc.). Of course, much of the research cited was based on work done with children who came from very traditional tribal backgrounds, and most was done 20 to 30 years ago. It is quite possible that you will not have any problems with learning differences.

Some of you might expect to have some difficulty adapting to taking medical histories and performing physical examinations on patients. Learning to communicate with patients from a different culture can be very challenging. You have to ask a number of personal questions when you take a medical history from a patient, and this is likely to make you uncomfortable. We consider this type of information to be the "property" of the patient, and it can be considered improper to ask for this property. Performing a physical examination can be even more difficult, because of many taboos and restrictions on the touching of individuals (other than one's family). Certain tribes dress very modestly, and so asking a patient to disrobe or performing a physical examination can prove to be traumatic (Alvord, 1997, p. 224).

In addition, individuals in some tribes do not discuss certain topics. In my own tribe, the Navajo, people do not talk about death—the eventuality of death, the possibility of imminent death, or the previous death of another. This is associated with a belief in the power of the spoken word and the concept that once something is "spoken into existence," the chances increase that whatever is spoken will have a higher likelihood of occurring. It is difficult for physicians who are raised with these concepts to explain to patients the possibility of future adverse outcomes or to address the issues associated with advance directives. Likewise, certain tribes, Navajo in particular, have cultural beliefs that do not allow them to touch dead bodies (Reichard, 1949).

This has caused problems for students in anatomy lab, when cadavers are dissected and in the hospital when patients expire. Some of you may have difficulty dealing with these issues. Students who come from more traditional backgrounds may need to undergo ceremonies of cleansing and purification after such encounters.

Obligations to Home Communities and Tribes

Many Native students have very strong ties to their culture and tribes. Families may request their presence at certain events of important social or religious significance. Some examples are the Lakota Sun Dance, Alaskan whale hunting seasons, and the Feast Days/Saint Days of the Southwestern Pueblo tribes. These fall out of sync with the usual "mainstream" American holidays. Obtaining permission to leave school to attend these events might prove to be difficult, particularly in the third and fourth years of medical school (the clinical years), as well as later in residency training. Those in charge (chief residents, attending professors) expect students to be present and participating at all times, except for grave emergencies. As a student, you may find yourself in a situation in which those around you have never even heard of your tribe's ceremonies. It becomes incredibly difficult to try to convince others of the importance of these events under such circumstances. Sometimes students will leave school without trying to explain, resigning themselves to face the consequences when they return. We strongly urge you not to do this but, rather, to use whatever resources you can to obtain permission to leave ahead of time. Individuals in the Office of Minority Affairs or other members of the faculty who you feel understand your background may be helpful advocates.

Ignorance About Native Americans and Native American Stereotyping by Mainstream American Society

Other problems that have arisen for Native American students who attend schools of higher education in non-Native communities occur as a result of misconceptions and stereotypes generated by American society. To this day, many Americans are unaware of the diversity and complexity of Native American tribes and communities or that hundreds of tribes exist, each with its own culture and language. Many believe that Native Americans still live in teepees, shoot bows and arrows, throw tomahawks, send smoke signals, say little other than an occasional grunt, wear beads and braids, and so on. The word *Indian* conjures up images of "red men" wearing feather headdresses. For example, the fact that Native Americans have had to endure being "mascots" for sports teams, with fans dressed in "war paint" and whooping "war cries" has caused Native people to question whether parts of American civilization will ever understand that it is wrong to stereotype another culture in this way. Many do not understand that this is a form of blatant racism and that it only underscores the profound degree of ignorance about Native people that still exists in America. As Garrod and Larimore (1997) write,

> Many Native Americans are unable to fathom why non-Native people fail to equate the use of Native Americans as mascots with unacceptable bigotry aimed at Blacks, Jews, or women. As has been pointed out time and again at Dartmouth and elsewhere, such hypothetical mascots as the "Washington White Trash," "Atlanta Niggers," and "Cleveland Jewboys" would simply not be tolerated today. (p. 9)

Native American students in higher education have many heartbreaking stories to tell.

> Bruce Duthu (Houma tribe) (1997) speaks of struggling with an "Indian symbol" mascot: "I was often put on the spot by students who wanted my opinion on the Indian symbol—specifically, why I found it offensive. One student wanted to know if there was a portrayal of Indian people that would be acceptable to us. In other words, "How can I still play Indian and not hurt your feelings?" (p. 239)

> Marianne Chamberlain (Assiniboine and Sioux) (1997) describes battling racism in college: "My work-study job was at the Dining Hall. The first month and a half of work went smoothly. Then one day, the student supervisor on duty approached me and asked if the rumor he had heard about me was true. 'They say that you are an Indian." I answered him honestly and told him, 'Yes, I am an American Indian.' 'Well, then,' he said, 'I better go and hide all the liquor. We don't want it to disappear or find you drinking on the job.' I could not believe what I was hearing. Then he continued, 'The only reason that you got into Dartmouth is because you are Native American. We all know that you are not smart enough to get in. They lower the standards for you people!' " (p. 158)

> Arvo Mikkanen (Kiowa/Commanche) (1997) writes: "I was constantly bombarded with myriad questions and statements from peers on every topic from the innocuous 'Does your mother wear

leather dresses?' to the often-repeated 'Did you know my great-grandmother was an Indian princess?' I remember vividly one incident when someone asked an Eskimo friend of mine whether he and his family lived in an igloo. I thought to myself, 'and these are supposed to be educated people.' " (p. 179)

Recently, I was asked by a college administrator if I spoke fluent "Native American"(!).

Likewise, most Americans are only vaguely aware of Native American history. A quick look at the American history books taught in most secondary schools prior to 1980 reveals a limited and often biased viewpoint. Like the slavery of Blacks and the internment of Japanese during World War II, America has had a hard time acknowledging the broken treaties and human rights abuses that occurred in the name of "Manifest Destiny." Consequently, Native students who enter non-Native communities to seek higher education find themselves dealing with many individuals who are ignorant about Native Americans and Native American history. Many students have told me they have found it psychologically exhausting to live in communities where so many individuals have no understanding of these issues.

Affirmative Action Backlash

Native American students, along with other underrepresented minorities, sometimes report that they encounter prejudice and feel unwelcome while at medical school, as a result of "affirmative action backlash." As Dr. Lois Steele (Assiniboine tribe) writes, "I had to prove that I was as good as everyone else. Some people felt I had gotten in (to medical school) because I am Indian and a woman" (Durrett, 1997, p. 93).

Secrets of Success for Native American Students

Native American students who are successful, like other students, tend to be highly motivated, intelligent, hardworking individuals who have already been successful in a premedical curriculum at the undergraduate level (or they would not have been considered for acceptance to medical school). You are students who, as undergraduates, have already learned to overcome the obstacles stated earlier, and you have started to prepare yourselves mentally for the rigorous curriculum demanded by medical school training. You are not afraid to seek out and ask for help when you need it. In addition, chances for success increase when families and communities are supportive. This frees students from some of the usual family obligations and allows them to concentrate more fully on medical school. Living too close to home can be a help or a hindrance: It can be helpful in that homesickness is lessened, but it can be a hindrance when it serves as a distraction, making it easy to return home for minor family problems or celebrations. In a similar vein, students who have stable family situations may tend to have less difficulty, because they will have less reason to return home for social or financial difficulties that arise from family matters. On the other hand, students who come from less stable environments may have developed extraordinary inner strength and adaptability that come from being self-sufficient.

The use of role models and mentors continues to be important. Because the absolute numbers of Native American physicians remains very small, it is quite likely that many of you will not have met a Native American physician. The Association of American Indian Physicians is a resource for students that serves many purposes: Among them, a mentor program has been established to give premedical and medical students access to Native physicians and to develop mentoring relationships. Additionally, this organization has established premedical workshops for premedical students to help them with the process of applying to medical school. Many students have found the discovery of a role model or mentor to be empowering, and this becomes very profound when a student meets a physician from his or her own tribe (many tribes still have only a handful of tribal members who are physicians). This helps students realize that becoming a physician is a real possibility rather than just a dream.

What Native Americans Offer the World of Medicine

Native American students remain relatively rare, and it is not unusual for some medical schools to lack a single Native student in their population. Because Native American physicians are also very rare, the most obvious asset that comes from training Native physicians is that it benefits Native American tribes and communities. Many Native physicians return to work in

Native American communities and are able to deliver a high level of care to patients as a result of the greater level of cultural understanding of patients. This commitment to patients is often an essential component of health care delivered by Native physicians. It can be very difficult to find non-Native physicians who are willing to deliver health care to Native American populations, particularly those who live in remote areas. Many physicians who work in tribal communities often have government contracts that provide loan repayment or other incentives. However, they frequently leave after spending one to three years in an area, and therefore long-term relationships with physicians are very rare for patients.

Traditional Native American perspectives on health are quite different from Western medical perspectives and offer many benefits that could be brought to the larger world's attention by Native American physicians.[1] For example, Native healers have never separated medicine and spirituality, believing that the two overlap substantially. Western medicine has only recently started to realize the importance of spirituality and mental health and how it relates to a patient's physical well-being. Many traditional healers also emphasize "preventive medicine" by advocating a lifestyle that is balanced. Spiritual health is considered essential. Exercise (or keeping one's body in good condition) and the avoidance of excessive eating or other indulgences are also necessary for balance. In other realms of life, many Native healers believe that good health for a patient also depends on the relationships that the patient has with his or her family and community. A person cannot be truly healthy unless his or her relationships are healthy as well. Therefore, a healer helps the patient, the family, and the community to determine deeper causes of stress and imbalance in a patient's life that may be causing or contributing to a physical problem. In addition, "living well" includes maintaining relationships with the animal world and the environment that are respectful and sacred. Because of the spiritual relationship to nature, the animal world and the environment have been protected and sustained for centuries prior to the arrival of Europeans to America. Since that time, the exploitation of animal and plant ecosystems and pollution of other elements of the environment (the air, land, and water) have gone unchecked until recent decades. The health of the human species depends on the existence of a healthy ecosystem, and Native American views may help reverse this disturbing trend.

The concepts described above demonstrate that Native ways of thinking can make substantial contributions to the world of medicine. Native American physicians who understand these approaches will offer benefit to patients and other health professionals with whom they work.

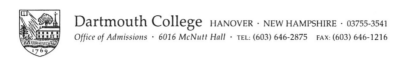

Dartmouth College HANOVER · NEW HAMPSHIRE · 03755-3541
Office of Admissions · 6016 McNutt Hall · TEL: (603) 646-2875 FAX: (603) 646-1216

To: _____
　　　FIRST　　　　　　MIDDLE　　　　　LAST NAME

From: Sylvia T. Langford, Director of Minority Recruiting

Since you have identified yourself as a Native American (American Indian, Alaska Native, and/ or Native Hawaiian), we encourage you to furnish us with the following information regarding your heritage. This information may be useful to us in working with the Bureau of Indian Affairs, Tribal Councils, and various Native American opportunity programs to identify additional financial aid resources for which you may qualify. Please complete and return this form as soon as possible.

Name: _____
　　　　　LAST　　　　　　　　FIRST　　　　　MIDDLE

Social Security Number: _____

Address: _____
　　　　　　STREET/BOX　　　　　　　CITY　　　　STATE　　ZIP

Telephone: Home ( ) _____ School ( ) _____

Tribe(s): _____

If Native Hawaiian, please list last Hawaiian surname in your family:

_____

Blood Percentage (full, ½, etc.):_____

Nearest Office of Hawaiian Affairs, Bureau of Indian Affairs Office, or Tribal Council Office in your area: _____

Does your school have a Native American Education Counselor? Yes_____   No_____
　　If yes, please list his/her
　　Name: _____ Title: _____
　　Telephone: ( ) _____

Do you maintain ties with any reservations, Hawaiian Homelands, or other Native American organizations or communities? Yes _____   No _____   If yes, please list
　　Name: _____ Address: _____

On the back of this form, please feel free to provide any additional information
that might help the Admissions Committee better understand and
evaluate your application with regard to your background and heritage.

NOTE

1. For discussions of Native American views of health, wellness, and spirituality, see the following: "Annie Kahn (Navajo Medicine Woman)" (1989), "Onandaga" (Lyans & Lyans, 1990), and *The Scalpel and the Silver Bear* (Alvord, 1999).

REFERENCES

Albuquerque Journal Navajo Times Albuquerque, NM Window Rock, AZ.

Alvord, L. A. (1997). Full circle. In A. Garrod & C. Larimore (Eds.), *First person, first peoples: Native American college graduates tell their life stories.* Ithaca, NY: Cornell University Press.

Alvord, L. A. (1999). *The scalpel and the silver bear.* New York: Bantam.

Annie Kahn (Navajo Medicine Woman). (1989). In B. Perrone, H. H. Stockel, & V. Krueger, *Medicine women, curanderas, and women doctors* (pp. 29-44). Norman: University of Oklahoma Press.

Appleton, N. (1983). *Cultural pluralism in education.* New York: Longman.

Association of American Medical Colleges, Division of Community and Minority Programs. (1996). *Minority students in medical education: Facts and figures X* (pp. 63, 67, 69). Washington, DC: Author.

Badt, K. L. (1995). *Charles Eastman: Sioux physician and author.* New York: Chelsea House.

Bazhonoodah, A. (1978). So long as this land exists, dark sky over black mesa. In P. Nabakov (Ed.), *Native American testimony.* New York: Penguin.

Biondel, R. (1980). American Indian education and confluent education: An overview of a case study. In American Indian Studies Center (Ed.), *American Indians in higher education.* Los Angeles, CA: Regents of the University of California.

Chamberlain, M. (1997). The Web of life. In A. Garrod & C. Larimore (Eds.), *First person, first peoples: Native American college graduates tell their life stories.* Ithaca, NY: Cornell University Press.

Durmont, R. (1972). Learning English and how to be silent: Studies in Sioux and Cherokee classrooms. In J. Cazden & D. Hymes (Eds.), *Function of language in the classroom.* New York: Teachers College Press.

Durrett, D. (1997). *Healers.* New York: Facts on File Books.

Duthu, B. (1997). The good ol' days, when times were bad. In A. Garrod & C. Larimore (Eds.), *First person, first peoples: Native American college graduates tell their life stories.* Ithaca, NY: Cornell University Press.

Erickson, F., & Mohatt, G. (1982). Cultural organization of participation structures in two classrooms of Indian students. In G. Spindler (Ed.), *Doing the ethnography of schooling.* New York: Holt, Rinehart & Winston.

Garrod, A., & Larimore, C. (1997). *First person, first peoples: Native American college graduates tell their life stories.* Ithaca, NY: Cornell University Press.

Havighurst, R. J. (1970). *National study of American Indian education.* Washington, DC: Office of Education.

Iverson, P. (1981). *The Navajo nation.* Albuquerque: University of New Mexico Press.

John, V. (1972). Styles of learning—Styles of teaching: Reflections on the education of Navajo children. In C. B. Cazden, V. P. John, & D. Hymes (Eds.), *Functions of language in the classroom.* New York: Teachers College Press.

Kleinfield, J. S. (1973). Intellectual strengths in culturally different groups: An Eskimo illustration. *Review of Educational Research, 43,* 341-359.

Kluckhohn, C. (1967). *Navajo witchcraft.* Boston: Beacon.

Lockhart, G. (1997). First morning light. In A. Garrod & C. Larimore (Eds.), *First person, first peoples: Native American college graduates tell their life stories.* Ithaca, NY: Cornell University Press.

Lyans, N., & Lyans, O. (1990). Onandaga. In S. Wall & H. Arden (Eds.), *Wisdomkeepers: Meetings with Native American spiritual elders.* Hillsboro, OR: Beyond Words.

Mikkanen, A. Q. (1997). Coming home. In A. Garrod & C. Larimore (Eds.), *First person, first peoples: Native American college graduates tell their life stories.* Ithaca, NY: Cornell University Press.

Ness, V. (1981). Social control and social organization in an Alaskan Athabaskan classroom: A microethnography of "getting ready for reading." In H. Trueba, G. Guthrie, & K. Au (Eds.), *Culture and the bilingual classroom* (pp. 120-138). Rowley, MA: Newbury House.

Phileon, W. E., & Galloway, C. E. (1969). Indian children and the reading program. *Journal of Reading, 12,* 598-602.

Reichard, G. (1949). The Navajo and Christianity. *American Anthropologist, 51,* 67.

Simmons, M. (1974). *Witchcraft of the Southwest.* Lincoln: University of Nebraska Press.

Wax, M., & Wax, D. (1964). Formal education in an American Indian community. *Social Problems, 11,* 95-96.

Wax, M. L. (1971). *Indian Americans: Unity and diversity.* Englewood Cliffs, NJ: Prentice Hall.

10 Focus on Mexican American Medical Students

MIGUEL A. BEDOLLA, MD, PHD, MPH

If one uses race[1] as a defining measure, Mexican Americans are difficult to classify. Although commonly called "Mestizos" (indigenous Indian, half Spaniard), the reality is much more complex. In the conquest of Mexico in the early 1500s, "White" Spaniards were accompanied by Black soldiers. By the middle of the 1700s, every settlement in what is now northern Mexico and the southwestern United States was made up of Spaniards, Blacks, and Indians. Inhabitants intermarried, resulting in, even within single families, enormous phenotypic diversity. These individuals were the ancestors of modern-day Mexican Americans. Today, Mexican Americans represent a fusion of cultural groups inhabiting the North American continent. Mexican Americans can appear to be White, Black, or Native American. Their diversity is reflected in their family surnames, which cannot be construed to necessarily reflect their ethnic identity: Mexican Americans have Spanish surnames such as Gonzalez and de la Garza, but there are also Mexican Americans with English, Irish, French, Belgian, German, Italian, Greek, Arabic, Jewish, Polish, Chinese, and Japanese surnames. Two of my colleagues, Drs. Fernandes and Alvares, are from India. At times, even the Mexican Americans themselves seem to be very confused about their own identifiers:

> I was interviewing a group of elderly Mexican Americans. At the end of the interview, I asked them to identify their ethnicity. One man immediately answered, "Mexican American," while a woman replied, "We are not Mexican Americans any more, we are Hispanic!"

Mexican Americans are now classified as Hispanic according to the Bureau of the Census. However, the terminology is still problematic. The common use of *Hispanic* seems (to many) to infer someone who is "neither White nor Black."

History of Mexican Americans in Medicine

The doors of U.S. medical schools were essentially closed to Mexican American applicants until the 1970s. Although a few students were educated in the United States, many older Mexican American physicians were educated in Mexico. Because anyone educated outside the United States is required to pass the Evaluation Commission of Foreign Medical Graduates (ECFMG) exam, Mexican American physicians, who had spoken English all their lives, were forced to pass a test demonstrating proficiency in the English language if they were to begin internships and residencies. In the United States, Mexican American physicians found themselves stigmatized as "foreign graduates," a code for "inferior." Numerous Mexican American friends and colleagues have told me that many residency programs, including some of the best in the country, refused to consider their applications, so they frequently ended up in positions that no one else wanted, in specialties they would not have selected, if they'd had the choice.

The doors of U.S. medical schools began to open for Mexican Americans in the early 1970s, although in 1982, U.S. medical schools enrolled only 278 Mexican American students in their combined freshman classes. This number represented 0.017% of the total U.S. freshman class that year. By 1995, the total number of Mexican Americans enrolled in the first year in all U.S. medical schools (primarily in California and Texas) had risen to 476, an increase of only 0.03% in 13 years. During the intervening years, the proportion of Mexican Americans in the *general* population of the United States grew to approximately 8% (in some South Texas areas, it approached 100%) (Association of American Medical Colleges [AAMC], 1996b, p. 17).

Although I am not aware of a single medical school that ever accepted a Mexican American who was not "qualified," it was perceived that the increase in the enrollment of Mexican Americans was a result of unfair implementation of the doctrine of affirmative action. It was commonly held that affirmative action had caused medical schools to lower their standards and to thus violate the civil rights of others, especially the rights of non-Hispanic White applicants. Anti-affirmative action campaigns in California and Louisiana resulted in two major setbacks to affirmative action: Proposition 209 (1996) in California and the *Hopwood* (1994) decision of the Federal Court in New Orleans (Academic Affairs, 1998). The *Hopwood* decision made it illegal for public universities within the jurisdiction of the New Orleans Court to consider race or ethnicity as a factor in admissions. It then extended to the state of Texas and included provisions against financial aid. The fact that State Attorney General Dan Morales[2] was a Mexican American seemed to cast an air of legitimacy to his support of the New Orleans Court decision.

The impact of anti-affirmative action efforts and resultant legislation was immediate. The number of Mexican American applicants and acceptances to medical school fell. Some students have indicated that because of anti-affirmative backlash, they believed access to financial aid to complete medical school would be denied them if they were accepted. To escape this backlash, many Mexican American students moved to states that they perceived would be more friendly than their home state.

Current Status

The size of the applicant pool has begun to rebound from anti-affirmative action attempts and legislation. In 1999, approximately 250 Mexican Americans were accepted to eight Texas medical schools from an applicant pool of 3,100 (AAMC, 1996a, pp. 1-4), approximately the same number who applied the year before the *Hopwood* Decision. This improvement is due in no small part to aggressive efforts by medical schools, the leaders being the University of Texas in Galveston and San Antonio, Baylor College of Medicine; the University of California, San Francisco (Fresno); and Stanford University. The University of Arizona, Tucson; University of New Mexico, Albuquerque; and the University of Illinois College of Medicine have also implemented aggressive efforts to recruit Mexican American medical students. Many schools have partnerships with regional universities to provide students with preliminary educational experiences so they can obtain competitive grade point average (GPA) and Medical College Admissions Test (MCAT) scores, the two pillars that support successful applications. Funding from the Division of Disadvantaged Assistance of the Bureau of the Health Professions of the Health Resources and Services Administration of the U.S. Department of Health and Human Services[3] has supported these schools' programs.

Special Challenges

A number of issues threaten the well-being of Mexican American medical students, as well as Mexican American faculty members at U.S. medical schools:

Mexican Americans Are "Foreigners"

The fundamental threat to the well-being of Mexican American medical students results from their being perceived as foreigners or the siblings of recent immigrants into the United States. They are never quite allowed to be just what they are: Americans. Some non-Mexican Americans are unsure whether Mexican Americans have the right to be there. Consider the following incident:

> Sometime after I joined the faculty of the medical school where I teach, I attempted to enroll my youngest children in the university's clinic. I was dressed in a white coat with the seal of the university. The coat had a name tag that clearly identified me as a university physician. When I asked how to enroll, the woman in charge only said, "Sir, are your children legally in the United States?"

This Mexican American man's family has resided in the State of Texas since 1750 and has played significant roles in the wars of the United States. Still, he was thought to be a foreigner.

This preceding situation is an example of a *microinsult,* a word I first heard during a presentation by the late Dr. Herbert Nickens, vice president of the Division of Community and Minority Programs of the AAMC. A microinsult is indirect; it insults by implication. Anyone who demonstrates anger after being targeted by a microinsult would seem to be overly sensitive. Microinsults take many shapes. It may be a blank stare at one's presence, a change in attitude, a condescending smile when pronouncing one's last name, or even the question "May I help you?" when help is not needed (the offer is used to put the person under the notice that he or she is being watched).

If you are a Mexican American interested in attending a medical school, you will have to learn to deal with microinsults, although it will be very difficult. Microinsults are always subtle and cowardly, and therefore very difficult to handle. They never quite seem to require a confrontation but can be very irritating and distracting. Thus, you will generally feel you have more to lose than win if you respond in a frontal attack to situations like these. The manifestation of anger does not seem appropriate; yet how do you handle microinsults? If overt anger is not appropriate, what then? A later section on "Microinsults in Medical School" offers some coping strategies for specific situations.

Cultural Concerns

Perhaps the most urgent cultural concern is based on demographics. Mexican American students will continue to come to medical school, and they will come in increasingly larger numbers. In a research project on the attitudes of ethnically diverse medical students, students were asked if they would be willing to abandon their ethnicity if that was necessary to become physicians. Mexican American male students said that they would rather be Mexican American than be physicians.

If you are afraid of losing your ethnic identity as you progress in your education, you may relinquish your course prematurely when challenged. Despite the possible implications of the preceding research question, you have to understand that medical education is not a threat to your ethnic identity. You cannot be other than what you are. You will still be what you are when you have finished your medical education. Go ahead, succeed!!

Microinsults in the Medical School

Few overt insults threaten your well-being as Mexican American students, but numerous microinsults will occur during the admissions process, in the classrooms, in the laboratories, in the wards of the hospital, and even in interactions with high-ranking administrators. Here are some rankling examples of what some students have encountered, with a follow-up discussion of coping strategies.

Admissions

The microinsult targeting Mexican Americans during the admission process is well typified in the following: Right after the *Hopwood* decision, I was invited to give testimony to the Texas Committee of the U.S. Commission on Civil Rights. A disturbing opinion was voiced numerous times by some of the members of the committee during the hearing in which I gave my testimony:

> Mexican Americans are not quite capable of meeting the standards for admission and dealing with the tasks of a professional education. Their culture does not push them toward success and is highly tolerant of failure. To bring them into medical school, standards will have to be lowered.

A microinsult illustrating the latter belief follows:

> It is interview day at a medical school. Applicants are seated randomly during lunch. A male non-Hispanic White is overheard telling a Mexican American female in a quiet, almost friendly voice: "I bet that your qualifications are not as good as mine and that you are only being interviewed because you are Hispanic."

Another form of microinsult targeting Mexican Americans has to do with language:

> A Mexican American applicant introduces himself to a non-Hispanic White interviewer. The interviewer responds in Spanish. The applicant tells the interviewer that although he is Hispanic, he does not speak Spanish. The interviewer is displeased and asks, "What kind of Hispanic are you who does not even know Spanish?!" The student never fully regains his confidence during the rest of the interview.

This example supports the contention that Mexican Americans are perceived as foreigners or recent immigrants: a foreigner or recent immigrant would speak what is considered a mother tongue.

A third type of microinsult during admissions occurs when the target is not even present:

> The admissions committee of a medical school is reviewing the application of a well-qualified Mexican American applicant from a family with a low income. When the chairman of the committee learns that she wants to become a neurosurgeon, he mockingly remarks, "So much for the interest of Mexican Americans to serve the underserved."

This classic example demonstrates that Mexican American medical students are expected to choose primary care careers and go back to their own communities (implied: where they belong).

The Classroom

Microinsults occurring in classrooms are often presented as bona fide educational experiences. One example comes from a teacher who presents Mexican Americans as a "race" in the process of "acculturation." The process of acculturation is generally presented as posing a threat to the health of Mexican Americans, as seen in the following:

> A professor presented the results of a study (of a Mexican American female patient) that compared the speed of gastric emptying after the ingestion of a "mainstream American diet, versus what the lecturer called a 'Mexican American diet.' The patient's stomach emptied faster with the mainstream American diet than with the Mexican American diet. The pancreas was not ready to secrete its insulin when the stomach emptied. Therefore, according to the professor, eating a mainstream American diet causes the high incidence of diabetes mellitus among Mexican Americans.

The implication: The best thing for Mexican Americans is to remain Mexican American.

On the other hand, some professors teach that Mexican Americans harbor diseases that are difficult to treat and that represent a threat to the rest of the American population:

> A pharmacology instructor was discussing resistance to antibiotics, saying that a particular type of resistance arises from the improper use of antibiotics. She goes on to describe what she believes to be antibiotic-prescribing patterns of physicians in Mexico, which

according to her, are so inadequate that they have caused the emergence of antibiotic resistant microbial strains. She continues, claiming that Mexicans carry these antibiotic resistant strains across the border and endanger the U.S. population. She closes with the comment, "Maybe we should shoot every Mexican that crosses the border." When the lone Mexican American student expresses his anger at the statement, she feigns not to understand why he is upset.

Mexican American patients are also presented, in subtle ways, as deviant and incapable of adhering to recommendations of health care providers:

A professor of obstetrics, talking to a class about weight gain during pregnancy, delivers a detailed lecture, including the diet the patient should follow. He adds, "Of course, all your time is wasted because your patients will go home to eat tacos!"

One of the most pernicious forms of insult is that which directly, but subtly, demeans Mexican American students:

A group of female medical students are conducting an experiment in one of the school's laboratories. After the third time that a male non-Hispanic White student comes over to ask what seems to be a trivial question, one of the students tells the only Mexican American in the group, "I wonder which one of us he is trying to get to know, because he certainly would not date a Mexican American like you."

In this case, the student at least expressed her belief. In most instances, beliefs go unexpressed. Even highly "acculturated" Mexican American students end up feeling isolated by the absence of a sense of real camaraderie, a camaraderie that helps a student succeed as a medical student.

The Wards and Other Clinical Sites

Microinsults that occur in the wards are similar. They insult Mexican American students indirectly by targeting Mexican American patients:

A surgical team arrives at the bed of a Mexican American patient where they discover that the patient speaks no English. The patient needs to have his wounds dressed; the chart clearly states that he must be anesthetized during this procedure. The surgeons decide that, because the patient cannot express himself in English, they will not anesthetize him. While dressing his wounds, they cause the patient to grimace in pain, then belittle him in front of the students.

A Mexican American patient has put images of saints on the wall of the ward. During rounds, a non-Hispanic medical student makes a series of remarks about how superstitious Mexican Americans are because they believe in saints and pray to them. Then she turns to the only Mexican American in the group and says, "But I know that you are not like that, Enrique."

The team is seeing a middle-aged Mexican American patient who speaks no English. He suffered orchitis as a young man and is sterile. His skin is thin and finely wrinkled. His body fat has a gynecoid distribution and the growth of hair on his forehead is abnormal. He is a hard worker and has been married for many years. When the attending asks about the patient's diagnosis, the resident replies, "Diabetes Type II. That is what all Mexicans have." Then the whole team begins to discuss the fact that the patient has been married for many years and tries to figure out how the patient makes love to his wife or how he keeps her happy.

Microinsults occurring on the wards are also aimed directly at the Mexican American medical students:

A third-year student wants to better understand what is going on with her patient. She asks a question. The resident leading the team responds, "What did you say your board score was?"

Administrative Employees

The medical school has a multitude of employees, ranging from the dean and his or her staff to the police force and custodians, some of whom believe that Mexican American students are guilty until proven innocent:

Tony is a first-year medical student, studying late in one of the labs of the medical school. When he finally leaves the campus, he realizes that he is being followed by the police. He begins to feel anxious because the policeman continues to follow him well after he has left the school grounds. Several miles after entering the expressway, the policeman finally signals Tony to pull over. He walks over to Tony's car and asks, "What were you doing at the medical school?" Tony says, "I was studying; I am enrolled there." The policeman says, "Mexicans don't study medicine. What were you stealing?"

You may also feel that many of the administrators whom you could ask for assistance are themselves perpetrators of microinsults:

A high-ranking officer of an academic health science center located in a region where a significant proportion of the population is Mexican American has invited a number of the employees of the center to a luncheon to celebrate their birthdays. One of them is a Mexican American faculty member. The officer begins to expound on the issues that the center is dealing with, one of which is the small number of Mexican Americans accepted to the center's medical school. He compares their numbers with the numbers of Asian Americans that have been accepted but neglects to explain the effect of social class and family income. He ends his presentation by saying, "If Asian Americans can [do well enough to get accepted] I don't see why Blacks and Mexican Americans can't."

Secrets of Success

About 95% of Mexican American students accepted graduate from medical school, most of them in four years, and some of them are being selected into the best residency programs around the nation. What are the secrets of their success?

First and foremost they are committed to succeed.

Jaime comes from a middle-income Mexican American family in South Texas. He excelled in athletics and attended a prestigious university on a football scholarship. After college, he was drafted into the professional football league where he played for several years and became extremely interested in treating facial injuries. To train for this, he left professional football and enrolled in dental school. By the end of his dental education, he realized that he would also need to complete medical school to be able to care for facial injuries most effectively. So he went to medical school. After medical school, he completed the training to become a plastic surgeon and a head and neck surgeon. Altogether, beyond college, he had about 14 years of medical and dental training. Soon after he finished his training, he became the head of the Department of Plastic Surgery at a medical school.

What is the secret of Jaime's success? The secret, I believe, is that he had a goal, the commitment to work toward its achievement and the discipline to work methodically. He has become one of the outstanding surgeons at his institution.

Draw strength from your commitment. Do not be distracted by the microinsults that you will no doubt encounter. Unpublished work of Dario Prieto, formerly of the AAMC, suggests that students who can deal with racism by staying focused on their commitment to succeed have a greater chance of succeeding (D. Prieto, personal communication, on various occasions). Roy P. Benavides, who won the Congressional Medal of Honor in Vietnam, used to say, "Quitters never win and winners never quit" (Christenson, 1998). Be a winner, stay focused, don't let the racism stop you.

The *second factor* that plays a role in the success of Mexican American medical students is the support they get from groups they organize or join. The students of San Antonio's Medical School began many years ago what eventually became the Texas Association of Mexican American Medical Students (although to be more inclusive, they were asked to change the name of their association to the Texas Association of Latin American Medical Students). Make an effort to identify a formally organized group of students who will understand your irritation, support you, and share with you the manner in which they deal with these situations.

The *third success factor* is your family. A student once told me that his grandfather, who owned a small ranch near Laredo, had set aside a few steers to sell when he was in need of money to complete his medical education. And another student, one of the most successful Mexican American medical students I have known, always enjoyed the support of not just his immediate family but of his extended family as well. The whole family took an enormous pride in his accomplishments. So when you find yourself attempting to deal with stressors, be creative; do not put yourself at risk by reacting inappropriately, and think of all those members of your family who are counting on you to make it through medical school and become a doctor. Again, Dario Prieto's unpublished research and my own experiences suggest that the Mexican

American students more likely to succeed are those who stay in touch with their families.

The *fourth factor* that plays a role in the success of Mexican American students is the support they obtain from a few, unique, medical school administrators.[4] These administrators have demonstrated a very clear commitment to recruiting and retaining Mexican American students into their medical schools. Take some time to identify these people. Ask your classmates who enrolled in the medical school before you. You can rely on their opinions and on the "grapevine" in which these opinions circulate. Students always know who will likely "go to bat for them" when they need it. Introduce yourself to that person. He or she does not have to be a Mexican American. Be open and be willing to experiment at finding someone with whom you can build a mentoring relationship.

The *fifth factor* that plays a role in your success is your skill in identifying the minimum amount of financial aid you'll need for medical school and to use the aid wisely. Plan your finances. Do not accept a loan just because it is offered to you. A loan is actually your future income, and the interest is what you are charged for using today the income that you have not yet earned. Bear in mind that you will have to pay the loan back, and with the interest, so keep your school debt at a minimum. Use the money to finance your education, not your standard of living. Become a Spartan. After all, medical school lasts only four years. Enjoy your income when you earn it.

The *sixth factor* that plays a role in the success of Mexican American medical students is the existence of programs funded to ensure your success (such as the Division of Disadvantaged Assistance of the Bureau of the Health Professions of the Health Resources and Services Administration of the U.S. Department of Health). The division's leaders have shown an unwavering commitment to implement the intentions of the U.S. Congress to increase the number of minority physicians. The division has funded programs such as the Health Careers Opportunities Program, and the Hispanic Centers of Excellence Program. Millions of dollars from these sources and from private foundations such as Kellogg, Robert Wood Johnson, and Howard Hughes have allowed many Mexican Americans to go through experiences that enabled them to be accepted into competitive medical schools. Find out which of the schools to which you are applying have programs that have been funded to promote your success. Do not be embarrassed to apply for their support. Our nation needs you to succeed. That is why our government and our nation's private foundations have funded these programs.

What Mexican Americans Offer
the World of Medicine

Traditionally, in Mexican American culture, humans are seen not as isolated, self-determined beings, but as members of a family. All the family participates in making decisions that Americans of many other ethnicities make alone. I worked with four generations of a Mexican American family while making the decision to disconnect or not to disconnect one of its members from a respirator. This supportive context is a valuable model for health care delivery.

A contribution noted by my non-Mexican American colleagues lies in attitude toward work. The perspective of many Mexican Americans is that they do not work for a company; they work for a person. They do not work for Outback Corporation; they work for Mr. Jackson, at Outback Corporation. The world of Mexican Americans is a world of persons. As physicians and other providers come more and more to work for health care corporations, the conditions are created in which it is easy to forget that the patient who is cared for is a person. Mexican American physicians can contribute to maintaining the personal aspect of medicine—keeping American medicine focused on service to the patient, not the corporation.

NOTE

1. When reviewing the historical records on "race," it becomes clear that race is not a scientific concept but an idea rooted in theology and adopted by politicians. The current meaning of race emerged within the context of the struggle for power within modern states, when politicians linked race to Manifest Destiny; that is, some (races) had a manifest destiny to dominate others (Crisp, 1995). There are scientists and politicos who continue to attempt linking race to biological foundations to this day.

2. Morales Letter Opinion LO97-001, Texas Attorney General, Dan Morales, February 5, 1997.

3. The past chief, Clay Simpson, and its chief at the time of this writing, Ciriaco Gonzalez, and their respective staffs have been especially supportive.

4. Several administrators of this type come to mind: From my own experience, Dr. Leonard E. Lawrence and Dr. Miguel Medina of the San Antonio Medical School, Dr. Billy Ballard of the Galveston Medical School, Dr. James Phillips of the Baylor Medical School, Dr. Catherine Flores of the San Francisco Medical School, Dr. Fernando Mendoza of the Stanford Medical School, Dr. Andrew Nichols and Carmen Garcia-Downing of the Tucson Medical School, Dr. Roberto Gomez of the New Mexico Medical School, and Dr. Jorge Girotti of the Chicago Medical School.

REFERENCES

Academic Affairs Human Resources. (1998). *Implementation of Proposition 209: How it impacts UC's employment practices.* University of California Office of the President. http://www.ucop.edu/humres/humres/policies/sp-2.html

Association of American Medical Colleges. (1996a). *Issue focus: Affirmative action in medicine.* Washington, DC: Author.

Association of American Medical Colleges. (1996b). *Minority students in medical education: Facts and figures* (Vol. IX). Washington DC: Author.

Christenson, S. (1998, November 8). Veteran faces new struggle: Medal of Honor recipient battles illness. *San Antonio Express-News* [San Antonio, TX], p. 1b. [Quoted material reprinted with permission. Copyright 2000, the San Antonio Express-News]

Crisp, J. E. (1995). Race, revolution and republic. In J. G. Dawson III (Ed.), *The Texas military experience: From the Texas Revolution through World War II* (pp. 32-48). College Station: Texas A&M University Press.

Hopwood v. Texas (861 F. Supp. 551 W.D. Tex. 1994).

11 Focus on Puerto Rican Medical Students

MARIA SOTO-GREENE, MD
JUAN C. MARTÍNEZ, EDD

As a Puerto Rican and native speaker of Spanish, you fall into the Hispanic category used by the U.S. Bureau of the Census. Mainland Puerto Ricans comprise the second largest Hispanic subgroup in the United States. Besides country of origin and diverse physical appearance, Hispanics differ in religious beliefs, political affiliation, diet, and region of residence (most Puerto Ricans live in the Northeastern United States). The reasons for living in this country also differ from group to group among the Hispanic community. The varying extent of acculturation makes this group even more heterogeneous (Harry, 1992).

Your membership within the Puerto Rican community is unique. The political association between the United States and Puerto Rico, which is quite different from other Hispanic American subgroups, allows travel between Puerto Rico and the mainland without particular documentation (Prewitt-Diaz, 1994). Although you might never have been to Puerto Rico, you nevertheless consider yourself a Puerto Rican and are very proud of your heritage. You may feel 100% Puerto Rican even when your heritage has been acquired only through your parents' ancestry.

History of Puerto Ricans in Medicine

You are among those who are still establishing the tradition of Mainland Puerto Ricans pursuing American medicine as a profession. The Association of American Medical Colleges (AAMC) first began collecting data on Puerto Ricans in 1973-1974. Earlier records indicate that in 1968, only three Puerto Ricans matriculated in U.S. medical schools. According to the AAMC (1999b), 30 years later, there were 106 Mainland Puerto Rican new entrants to the class of 1998 (the data refer to entrance and not completion rates, which also have been lower for minorities when compared with Whites). Also noteworthy is the low representation of Puerto Rican physicians as medical school faculty members. AAMC data in 1997 indicate that there were only 674 Puerto Rican faculty physicians employed in all medical schools, including Puerto Rico (AAMC, 1999a).

Current Status

The AAMC has divided Puerto Ricans into Mainland and Commonwealth applicants. Mainland Puerto Ricans are defined as those who reside in the United States and who, based on their number in the U.S. population, are underrepresented in the medical profession. Commonwealth Puerto Ricans are defined as those who live and have been educated in Puerto Rico. However, the migration patterns of Puerto Ricans make it difficult to fully categorize applicants. Because many Mainland Puerto Ricans are considered underrepresented in U.S. medical schools, the pool for recruitment and enrollment is limited. Similar to other ethnic groups in the United States, some Puerto Ricans have joined the ranks of the middle and upper classes. As a result, the profile of Puerto Rican applicants has changed somewhat, and medical schools' admissions committees have begun to question their eligibility as underrepresented group candidates. Despite the fact that some Puerto Rican applicants' parents may have achieved college education, they are often the first to have done so in the family and do not necessarily have enough experience with the academic system to give their children more than a socioeconomic advantage.

Unfortunately, low Medical College Admission Test (MCAT) scores and grade point averages (GPAs) diminish opportunities for admission to medical school for many Puerto Rican students. The AAMC 1996 and 1997 MCAT Performance Reports indicate that among U.S. Hispanics, Mainland Puerto Ricans achieved the lowest scores in each test category. The Puerto Rican candidate's number of science courses taken, GPA, previous medical exposure, and MCAT scores achieved may be lower than their majority peers. Although the myth is that minority students are not capable of performing well in standardized examinations, a substandard showing may result from poor educational preparation. In addition, their lack of exposure and practice on this type of test contribute to low scores, especially because limited financial resources prohibit some students from enrolling in costly commercial MCAT review courses.

In essence, minority physicians continue to be vastly underrepresented in the nation's workforce. Over 80% of the estimated 737,764 physicians in the United States are White, approximately 11% are Asian, and about 5% are Hispanic (U.S. Bureau of Labor Statistics, 1998, p. 178). Significant changes will not be achieved if minority medical school matriculants continue to experience decreased acceptance to medical school. In fact, the total number of underrepresented minority matriculants fell to 1,762 in 1997, the lowest since 1991 (AAMC, 1999b).

Special Challenges

What Have We Faced to Get Here?

Now that you are a medical student, you have found that the challenges facing you are different from those you faced at the undergraduate college level. What you considered very hard work then now seems easy compared with medical school demands. Indeed, you worked hard to maintain a good college GPA while completing medical school applications, getting your letters of reference in order, and preparing for the MCAT. In addition to all that, very likely you were holding a job. You were one of the few Hispanics applying to medical school and perhaps the only Puerto Rican. When you look around your school, you may see that you are one of the few (if not the only) Puerto Ricans accepted into your class.

The U.S. Hispanic population is rapidly growing. It is estimated to become the largest minority group in the United States by the year 2005, and by the year 2050, it is projected that one of every five Americans will be Latino (Health Resources and Services Administration, 1998; U.S. Bureau of the Census, 1998). Then why the small number of Puerto Ricans in medical school? Some of the answers may lie in poverty-stricken school settings, the challenges of juggling two cultures, increased mobility, language differences, educators' negative responses, and high dropout rates.

The most visible reason for lower numbers of Puerto Ricans at the end of the educational pipeline is *poverty*. In common with many U.S. minority children, a large number of Puerto Ricans attend segregated schools, which are located in poor school districts with many crowded classrooms and poor counseling services (Meléndez, 1985). The American Council on Education reports that, similar to African Americans, a higher percentage of Hispanic families have incomes below poverty level. Among U.S. Hispanics, poverty continues to be a serious problem for Puerto Ricans (Reed & Ramirez, 1998). Puerto Rican children are more likely than other Hispanic children to live in urban settings in low-income, female-headed families (U.S. Bureau of the Census, 1998). Poverty is known to place children at an educational disadvantage (McMillen, Kaugman, & Klein, 1997).

Since your first day in the U.S. school system, you were classified as an ethnic minority. For many members of minority groups, acculturation is seen as the means to blunt the conflicts that cross-cultural interactions often present. However this *acculturation has not been easy*. Studies indicate that for Mexican Americans and Puerto Ricans, the level of acculturation has been diminished by the geographical proximity maintained to the traditional culture (Laung, 1988; Morales, 1986; Ramirez & Castaneda, 1974). Puerto Ricans frequently relocate between the island and the mainland. Indeed, in 1985, the largest number of students entering and leaving New York City schools within the same academic year were from Puerto Rico (Cohen, 1995). Therefore, *mobility* often has a negative effect on students' academic achievement, especially among low-income minority students. A different language and cultural experience at each end of the migration stream compounds the problem, interrupting the educational process by frequent travel between island and mainland U.S. schools. As a result, children experience confusion and frustration, which frequently has a negative impact on their education and school performance (Cohen, 1995).

Another acculturation challenge affecting your academic progress is the task of juggling home and school cultures. Schools, while providing an education, most definitely affect the way in which students see themselves and others in the world around them. Different from many other Hispanic Americans, you most likely were born in the mainland United States or arrived here when you were very young. Although you are an American citizen, you may strive to maintain your identity as a U.S. Puerto Rican and *struggle to maintain your home values and beliefs* within a school setting. For example, a Puerto Rican may be taught at home not to make direct eye contact when spoken to by an individual perceived to be an authority figure, whereas American schools expect direct eye contact in most interactions. In college, culturally speaking, you might have found difficulty in expressing disagreements with your professors' views. This is in some part due to Hispanic students' tendency to not actively challenge the teacher or to reserve judgment out of respect for an authority figure. Hispanic students also favor a cooperative orientation rather than being competitive, which creates conflict in the mainstream classroom where a competitive orientation is usually the norm. Children of Hispanic culture have been taught not to promote themselves over their peers. Unfortunately, this behavior might be misjudged as linguistically or cognitively limited, underprepared or lacking in initiative, easily intimidated, or arrogant (Smith, 1989). Your being frequently misjudged may lead you to feel very different from members of the majority group and conflicted in your identity and self-esteem.

Your *language* skills also might have been an issue throughout your education. It is almost certain that you spoke Spanish before English. Once in school, the frequent use of English made you fluent in a second language. At least one of seven people in this country grew up or will grow up speaking a language other than English (Barringer, 1993). Not understanding that English is your second language, your teachers may have maintained that you had reading problems and, possibly, a learning disability. Every year, a disproportionate number of U.S. Hispanic children are diagnosed as learning disabled. A study conducted in Los Angeles showed that teachers routinely categorized their students as fast or slow learners as early as the first two weeks of first grade. Because the U.S. educational system uses a monocultural curricular content, students who are native speakers of languages other than English are at a disadvantage and as a result are frequently misdiagnosed as having a disability.

An individual's values, beliefs, and behaviors create rich differences among human beings. Hispanics are no exception. Educators' lack of understanding and/or training about a group's history and culture, coupled with the school's inadequate curricula, contribute to a negative experience for many Puerto Rican youngsters. As Hispanic medical school educators, we find that these previous *negative educational experiences* contribute to a student's self-image and his or her tendency not to seek the advice of counselors. These same processes may have affected your high school and college experiences. How learners feel about the setting they are in, the respect they receive from the people around them, and their ability to trust their own thinking and experience, powerfully influence their concentration, imagination, effort, success, and willingness to continue. Students who feel unsafe, disconnected, and disrespected are unlikely to be motivated to learn (Wlodkowski & Ginsberg, 1995). Puerto Ricans tend to see life as a network of personal relationships and become uneasy when they must rely on impersonal interactions rather than personal relationships (Fitzpatrick, 1987). Educators who see them as passive, conforming, and trusting misunderstand the culture. People's motivation to learn is directly connected to a vision of a hopeful future (Courney, 1991; Ogbu, 1987). If there is no vision of the future, there will be no motivation to learn. Perhaps this is why so many of your high school and even college classmates become discouraged and disinterested.

The *high dropout rate* among Hispanics has tremendously reduced the number of Puerto Ricans who could aspire to a college education (McMillen et al., 1997). The number of Hispanics attending college and attaining a degree continues to be disproportionately low compared with White students (Reed & Ramirez, 1998). Socioeconomic status, schools attended, language difficulties, and the "learning disabled" label that has been attached to a high number of Puerto Rican students are among the reasons why students fail to compete at the university level (Anderson, 1988).

Findings thus far serve to support the hypothesis that Puerto Rican students who have successfully gained entry into medical school have overcome major obstacles. These obstacles, which range from poor academic preparation in secondary schools, poverty, and mobility, coupled with a lack of guidance and a lack of role models, impede their opportunity for academic success.

Medical School Challenges

Isolation

You may feel isolated in medical school. Most of your friends and peers disappeared along the educational pipeline. You are pursuing a career that traditionally limits access to U.S. Puerto Ricans. Throughout this time, you have encountered differing values between those at home and in school, which are disorienting and perhaps contribute to a poor self-image.

Choosing Between Medicine and Family Commitments

In common with other Hispanics, Puerto Rican students usually maintain a strong commitment to their family. This is best illustrated in the personal thoughts and experiences shared by "Adan" who relates the following:

For an individual just arriving in the United States from Puerto Rico, there are numerous obstacles he must overcome, the most traumatic of which is to surrender language, tradition, and family values in order to assimilate. For those unwilling to surrender even the most trivial part of their identity, the cauldron is extremely unforgiving. Those willing to compromise the values and ethics of their culture in favor of the American culture will find the road to success and achievement a much smoother endeavor and easier to maneuver.

Adan's feelings are similar to those of many Puerto Ricans who migrated to the United States. Yet why should this be so if they are American citizens by birth? He continues:

For someone, like myself, who is born and raised within the Puerto Rican tradition, the experience is equally traumatic. My rearing was quite traditional with Spanish as my primary language, the Puerto Rican culture and value system, and the Puerto Rican family hierarchy. The South Bronx was my home for over 20 years. I was educated there, had friends there, and my family still calls it home. Growing up, the concept of "respect" was drilled into me from birth. Respect elders, respect prominent people, respect those in authority, and respect the place you are in and the people you are with. In certain instances, it is even appropriate to stifle yourself and hold your thoughts ("hold your tongue") when interacting with the people you are supposed to respect. In the workplace, you are supposed to do a job well and not strive toward upward mobility. Promotions and achievements are not thought of as part of the normal ascent through the system but, rather, a gift from someone in authority. When in need, the typical Puerto Rican is supposed to be capable of solving his or her own problems. For me, it was even more difficult as an only child. Family illness was my first real problem. My father had a major stroke, which led to a yearlong hospitalization. He was, and still is, a stubborn Puerto Rican male who cannot (or will not) accept help from others. This refusal for rehabilitation care has left him hemiplegic. Today, my mother looks after all his needs, for it would be a cultural sin to place him in a nursing home to be cared for by strangers. And so, here I am, an only son, taking responsibility for my parents and navigating my way through medical school.

Concerns when I reentered academics focused on my responsibilities to my family. The "what happens if?" question is quite prominent. What shall I do if? Who can I turn to? These questions, and
many others, persist as I enter my third year of medical education.

While not entirely unique to Puerto Rican students, Adan's experience is
illustrative of the importance given to family values. He exemplifies a sense
of frustration in the "machismo" behavior of his father, the role his mother
must continue to assume, and the concept of respect for others even when
their viewpoints clearly differ.

Finances

Financial aid is critical for most Hispanics who need to obtain it to complete medical school. Interviews with Hispanic high school, college, and medical students always contain two major issues. The first is their fear of heavily
relying on financial aid, and second is their ability to navigate through the
financial nightmare that the process entails. Their educational debt increases
if they feel the need to actually use their academic financial aid to alleviate
family monetary woes (see Chapter 7).

Lack of Encouragement From the Educational System

Throughout their education, minority students often encounter individuals
who have made them feel as if they were destined for failure. This situation
has most likely given them the feeling that medicine is a dream fulfilled only
by an exceptional few. When you first expressed your interest in medicine as a
profession, you might have been told "you can't succeed in medical school
because you just don't have what it takes educationally or intellectually."
These humiliating and discouraging comments are based on a myth undermin-
ing the intellectual capabilities of minorities as a whole (see Chapter 5). The
paucity of faculty members and administrators able to understand the experiences that students of different cultures and linguistic groups have to face further exacerbates the problem.

Thus far, we have discussed many of the commonalities that Puerto Ricans
share with the other major ethnic minorities. At the same time, we have identified unique challenges faced by this group. As a Puerto Rican who has made it
to medical school, you must be feeling like one of the lucky or chosen few.
You are fortunate indeed to have overcome the filtering that occurs through-

out the educational pipeline. Underrepresentation of Puerto Ricans in medicine refers not only to medical students but also to medical school faculty, support staff, and administrators. To increase the presence of Puerto Ricans in the field of medicine, it is vital that the history and experience of this group in the United States be understood. Only this will provide a voice of change.

Secrets of Success and Survival

Keep focused on your academics and future professional interests. Do not become discouraged. It is important to make your viewpoints heard. To survive medical school demands, while contributing back to the community, some Puerto Rican and other Hispanic medical school students unite and share common issues and concerns. In 1972, medical school students in Boston and New York City founded the Boricua Health Organization (BHO). BHO was a direct response to the political climate existing at the time. BHO's main objective was to serve as an advocate for the rights of Hispanics in the United States. BHO's most pressing concerns were access to quality health care and the recruitment of Hispanics into health professions. By the late 1970s, BHO had established chapters in major northeastern cities. Now under the name of Boricua/Latino Health Organization (BLHO), this organization provides Hispanic and other minority students with a sense of unity and common goals. It also extends support to other Hispanic medical students with similar academic and personal experiences. The name was adapted to reflect the expanding diversity among the Hispanic population in the region. BLHO still serves to strengthen students' ambitions to one day become physicians who will serve the community.

The Student National Medical Association (SNMA) is another key organization for the minority medical student. In some schools, SNMA is the only organization available to minority medical students. It offers support as well as the opportunity for students to gain professional direction and understanding of the communities they will serve (see Chapter 8).

As a Puerto Rican student, you will need to learn how to strike a better balance between what has been taught by your parents and what is requisite to succeed in this complex educational system. By no means does this imply giving up cultural and family values and traditions. Rather, we must stress the development of additional coping strategies. For example, respect for authority figures, while important, should never compromise our making our points heard, loud and clear. By voicing our feelings and concerns, we challenge others to address our needs even if it means making an adjustment in their behavior to accommodate the normal human variation seen in American society.

What Puerto Ricans Offer the World of Medicine

As members of two cultures and as people possessing two languages, Puerto Ricans can offer an understanding of the values, language, cultural, and other factors that play a role in health care delivery to a diverse population. Although many would argue that as long as physicians provide quality care, their ethnicity is unimportant, minority patients will challenge physicians who lack knowledge about characteristic disease patterns, beliefs, customs, and concerns that are far different from those learned in medical school. Traditionally, Puerto Ricans have consulted "espiritistas" (spiritual healers) and "santeros" (folk healers) as part of their health care process. They also hold physicians in high regard. The literature on Hispanics indicates that it is the socially and economically disadvantaged group that is more skeptical and uninformed about seeking medical services. Yet there is a growing trend in the higher socioeconomic group to refrain from entrusting all health care decisions to physicians. Puerto Rican physicians are more likely to be knowledgeable about their culture and thus can help educate their colleagues, enabling them to provide more understanding care to Puerto Rican patients.

The premise that minority physicians, more than members of the majority group, serve predominantly minority communities was confirmed by a study recently conducted in California that analyzed physicians' data from 1990 (Komaromy et al., 1996). This study supports the unique role of African American and Hispanic physicians in the care of an underserved population. It raises concerns about the threat of dismantling affirmative action programs. Although most educators are fully aware that decisions have been made to end affirmative action programs in California and Texas, it is important not to lose sight of the ripple effect this may have across the nation.

Conclusion

Throughout this chapter, the educational, socioeconomic, and cultural challenges of the Puerto Rican population have been discussed. To continue to make a difference and provide an ethnically diverse physician workforce, it is important to recognize the unique issues faced by this very important community.

In closing, it is our very traditions that allow us to be caring, compassionate physicians with an ability to better understand the psychosocial needs of our patients. The best physicians are those who can couple their intellectual abilities with their attributes to make a lasting contribution to society. We, too, as Puerto Ricans should be able to attain such recognition.

Puerto Rican students must be active in seeking those who care and can assist them in realizing their full potential. Writing this chapter presented its challenges, because the literature available specific to Puerto Ricans is limited. Write about your experiences so that others can learn from them. Welcome the challenge of changing your life, your family, and future generations as you enter the medical profession.

REFERENCES

Anderson, J. (1988). Cognitive style and multicultural populations. *Journal of Teacher Education, 39*(1), 2-9.

Association of American Medical Colleges. (1999a). *Student and applicant information: FACTS—Applicants, matriculants and graduates.* Washington, DC: Author.

Association of American Medical Colleges. (1999b). *Publications and information resources: U.S. medical school faculty, 1997.* Washington, DC: Author.

Barringer, F. (1993, April 28). When English is a foreign tongue: Census finds sharp rise in 80's. *New York Times,* p. A-1.

Cohen, D. L. (1995, May-June). Family ties. *Teacher-Magazine, 6*(8), 18-19.

Courney, S. (1991). *Adults learn: Toward a theory of participation in adult education.* New York: Routledge, Chapman & Hall.

Fitzpatrick, J. P. (1987). *Puerto Rican Americans: The meaning of migration to the mainland.* Englewood Cliffs, NJ: Prentice Hall.

Harry, B. (1992). *Cultural diversity, families, and the special education system: Communication and empowerment.* New York: Teachers College Press.

Health Resources and Services Administration (HRSA). (1998). *Current population reports* (Bureau of Primary Health Care Uniform Data System, 1997). Washington, DC: Government Printing Office.

Komaromy, M., Grumach, K., Drake, M., Vranizan, K., Lurie, N., Keane, D., & Bindman, A. (1996). The role of Black and Hispanic physicians in providing health care for underserved populations. *New England Journal of Medicine, 334*(20), 1305-1310.

Laung, E. K. (1988, October). *Cultural and acculturation commonalities and diversities among Asian Americans: Identification and programming considerations.* Paper presented at the Ethnic and Multicultural Symposia, SIA, Dallas, TX.

McMillen, M., Kaugman, P., & Klein, S. (1997). *Dropout rates in the United States: 1995.* Washington, DC: Department of Education, National Center for Education Statistics.

Meléndez, E. (1985, Fall). Down the upstaircase. *Educational Record, 66*(4), 46-50.

Morales, J. (1986). *Puerto Rican poverty and migration.* New York: Praeger.

Ogbu, J. U. (1987). Variability in minority school performance: A problem in search of an explanation. *Anthropology and Education Quarterly, 18,* 312-335.

Prewitt-Diaz, J. O. (1994). *The psychology of Puerto Rican migration.* Lancaster, PA: Author.

Ramirez, M., & Castaneda, A. (1974). *Cultural demography, biocognitive development and education.* New York: Academic Press.

Reed, J., & Ramirez, R. R. (1998). *The Hispanic population in the United States: March 1997 (Update)* (pp. 20-511). Washington, DC: Department of Commerce, Economics and Statistics Administration.

Smith, D. G. (1989). *The challenge of diversity: Involvement or alienation in the academy?* (ASHE-ERIC Higher Education Report, No. 5). Washington, DC: Association for the Study of Higher Education.

U.S. Bureau of the Census. (1998). Health care uniform data system, 1997. *Current population reports.* Washington, DC: Government Printing Office.

U.S. Bureau of Labor Statistics. (1998). Employment and earnings. *Household data annual averages.* Washington, DC: Government Printing Office.

Wlodkowski, R. J., & Ginsberg, M. B. (1995). *Diversity and motivation: Culturally responsive teaching.* San Francisco: Jossey-Bass.

12 Managing Racism

KEVIN BAKEER AL-MATEEN, MD
CHERYL S. AL-MATEEN, MD

> Racism—The belief that race is the primary determinant of human traits and capacities and that racial differences produce an inherent superiority of a particular race.
>
> —*American Heritage Dictionary, Third Edition*

"He kept getting me confused with the previous month's student and making me responsible for assignments he had given her," she said. "When I was sick for three days, I called the senior resident, the surgery department, and the curriculum director; I still had to give him doctor's notes explaining my whereabouts."

These comments from a Black medical student describe her experience with the attending physician during a general surgery clerkship. Although not blatantly racist in form, she perceived his actions to be racially motivated because the White students were not treated the same way. Performance evaluations in your clinical clerkships are largely subjective. "Nonsurgical attitude," "nonteam player," "limited knowledge base," and "attitude problem" are common descriptions of medical student performance that could mask potentially racist feelings. Proving that racism is at the core of one's behavior is difficult. As the student above concluded, there may be situations that you perceive as racist but in which you feel at a loss for how to respond. Racism can be pervasive in the United States. It may be institutional or individual. Although blatant racial slurs, graffiti, or violent acts toward students are uncommon on medical school campuses, you may be faced with more subtle forms of prejudice.

In this chapter,[1] we explore the psychological roots of racism to help you understand what drives this behavior and its psychological effects on the victim. We will then discuss means of supporting your peers through these experiences. The options that may be available within your university to deal with racism and the importance of obtaining objective evidence to support your claims are emphasized. We stress that racism does not equal helplessness in your effort to be evaluated fairly. Armed with this information, you can devise prevention and intervention strategies to help you graduate with your self-esteem intact.

Historical Perspectives

It has been more than 135 years since Rebecca Lee became the first Black woman physician from an American medical school when she graduated from Boston's New England Female Medical College in 1864. Despite Dr. Lee's achievement at this predominantly White medical school, the majority of the nation's minority physicians are graduates of two historically Black medical colleges, Howard University and Meharry Medical College. By 1969, 75% of all Black medical students (3% of all medical students) were enrolled in these institutions (Association of American Medical Colleges [AAMC], 1987).

Federally and privately sponsored affirmative action programs, which sought student enrollments that matched general population racial percentages, raised minority representation in American medical schools to its first peak of 8.1% in 1975 (AAMC, 1997). Within a 10-year period, the historically Black college contribution to the minority physician population decreased to 20%. As affirmative action programs are eliminated, fewer students from underrepresented groups will be admitted. Because of often sparse representation of minorities on medical school faculties (Ellis, 1997), not only are you likely to be in a small cohort in your medical school class but also in your medical school community at large. As a result, you may feel more culturally isolated in racially sensitive situations. One study found that 76% of fourth-year minority medical students said that their race affected their educational experience, compared with 30% of White students. Asian students experienced the same difficulties, often to a higher degree (Bright, Duefield, & Stone, 1998). These students attended schools that had diverse student bodies. They cited difficulties in establishing a peer support network, establishing a good working relationship with peers, and finding same-race role models and mentors.

Understanding the psychological roots of racism and potential effects on psychosocial development helps you identify, confront, and even eliminate racial discrimination in your medical school.

Psychology of Racism

Racism can occur on an individual, institutional, or ubiquitous cultural basis (Winton, Singh, & McAleavy, 1998). *Individual racism* develops in relation to attitudes demonstrated by parents or is found in society at large. It can be revealed through thoughts or behaviors. *Institutional racism* also develops over time and can cause unfair restrictions on opportunity for certain groups of people. *Cultural racism* involves a combination of institutional and individual forms (Dovidio & Gaertner, 1986).

Discrimination is the behavior that results from prejudice and racism. People are prone to stereotype others based on easily identified characteristics such as race or culture. Once a stereotype is identified and repeated, it becomes "accepted." Racist jokes are examples of culturally accepted stereotyping and discrimination. When these ideas are not tested or questioned, they become the basis for interacting with those from the stereotyped group. Sadly, when individuals and institutions make decisions based on stereotyped misinformation, social reality becomes further distorted (Winton et al., 1998).

A range of behaviors can develop from racism. The most extreme forms of racism include genocide, ethnic cleansing, terrorism, murder, and other forms of physical attack. Destruction of property, graffiti, hate speech, and discrimination, although not physically harmful, all have a definite impact on the victim's psyche.

Many of these events can be classified as hate crimes. A *hate or bias crime* is usually an excessively brutal event committed by several perpetrators against an individual based on a global characteristic such as race. Such crimes psychologically affect the individual and the community, especially other members of the same group.

In medical school, you are most likely to encounter *hate or bias incidents*. These are episodes that may involve the use of "harmful words or actions motivated by prejudice against a person or property which do not fall into any criminal category" (McLaughlin & Brilliant, 1997, p. 13). If you find yourself the victim of such an incident, the absence of legal recourse is an emotionally intensifying factor.

One type of hate incident, *verbal assault or harassment,* is a symbolic form of violence, which reinforces the sense of being a vulnerable member of an ostracized group. Your sense of security is violated. You may try to minimize the effects of a verbal assault, but the resultant emotional scars are more difficult to recognize than physical wounds. In fact, your ability to minimize the situation may make it more difficult for you to understand any feelings of fear or self-hatred that you might experience. The lingering evidence of a physical assault can be a concrete springboard for understanding your emotional sequelae. Verbal assaults leave no such scars, so it may be difficult to understand why you feel so bad. If you are frequently verbally assaulted, you may restrict your behaviors and become isolated. Fear of physical harm after verbal assault can cause the same kind of isolation behaviors seen after a physical attack (Garnets, Herek, & Levy, 1990).

The incidence of bias events in medical schools has not been reported in the literature. However, racism on college campuses has been studied (Berrill, 1992).

Racism on Campus

"My medical school has an office to support minority . . . students," said Lauren. "We were all feeling the usual . . . strain. . . . Some Black students might ask for assistance and the director of the support office would arrange for a tutorial with a graduate student. My friend, who is Black, brought me to the tutorial. Several Black students confronted her, indicating that I was not welcome because I was not Black and was using resources not designated for me." Lauren is of Korean ancestry.

Race incidents can be majority versus minority, minority versus majority, or minority versus minority conflicts. A hostile racial climate can be created by students, teachers, or staff (Chun & Zalokar, 1992). Incidents can include jokes, slurs, posters, harassment, or intimidation (U.S. Commission on Civil Rights, 1990).

As colleges and medical schools become more culturally diverse, ignorance of cultural differences by the faculty, staff, and students should be unacceptable to your medical school's administration. Insensitive comments and behaviors in the medical school community are a result of society's failure to keep up with this change. As the size of any group enlarges beyond historical norms, demands on the institution for recognition of that group's unique needs are more likely to occur (U.S. Commission on Civil Rights, 1990). The fight for recognition between different minority groups can also lead to conflict.

People in the United States often oversimplify racial differences into a "Black versus White" dichotomy, neglecting other ethnic groups (Nebraska Advisory Committee, 1990). As student financial aid resources decrease and the number of groups that qualify increases, the competition for them escalates. Students unfamiliar with the history behind race or need-based financial aid may develop a perception of being discriminated against if they are disqualified because of race. Recognition by the majority population of the need to be culturally sensitive in our multicultural society is a recent event.

Impact on the Victim

Although *bias incidents* are generally not as severe as *bias crimes,* understanding the reactions to more severe incidents helps you recognize how you may respond to a less severe encounter. If you are a victim of hate violence, the most frequent emotional response is anger at the perpetrator. Other emotional responses include fear of injury or death, sadness, powerlessness, and suspicion (Barnes & Ephross, 1994). Your self-esteem will likely remain intact if you associate the incident with the perpetrator's prejudice and racism. If you see the incident as a result of blatant meanness and cruelty, you are more likely to risk developing erosion in your basic ability to trust others (Bard & Sangrey, 1979).

A difficult aspect of bias crime is that the victim usually recognizes that there was nothing that could have altered being vulnerable in the situation because it relates to a core aspect of the victim's identity (AAMC, 1987; McLaughlin, Brilliant, & Lang, 1995; Roberts, 1995). Race is an immutable aspect of your identity. This can heighten your sense of vulnerability and hopelessness. Such crimes are meant to send the message to the victim and others that fear and terror can follow at random.

Bias incidents affect members of groups frequently targeted for racist comments and behavior. They are reminded of their vulnerability and also feel victimized (McLaughlin et al., 1995). The message can be compounded if racist incidents are handled inadequately by your school's administration. You may lose your sense of belonging to the medical school community and nurture feelings of betrayal by the administration. The offender's actions may be misperceived as representative of institutional indifference.

Phases of Victim Reaction to Racist Incidents

There are several phases to a victim's reaction to a racial bias crime or incident (Bard & Sangrey, 1979; Sales, Baum, & Shore, 1984). During the *impact phase,* you may need crisis intervention from a mental health professional. This person will assess and help you to contact your coping resources. For common or less severe incidents, use your established support network of family and friends.

The next phase is the *recoil phase.* If a serious crime has occurred, the counselor or therapist will continue to support you. As a survivor of such an incident, you need to ventilate your feelings of horror and terror, express anger toward your assailants in a constructive manner, and work toward understanding the incident in terms of the global aspects of hatred that the perpetrator represents. Self-defense classes may help you direct your anger. Finally, report the event to law enforcement or university administration officials if warranted.

During the final *reorganization stage,* a therapist's goal is to help you integrate the traumatic experience into your worldview. If you experience a relatively minor incident, the stages described above will likely occur in a less intense manner.

Intervention Strategies

"On my pediatrics rotation, we were required to turn in patient write-ups. The attending simply wrote check marks on all of the papers turned in by the other students. However, on mine he would write comments like 'poor grammar' or 'wrong use of word' in red ink throughout the paper." The attending said, "Your fund of knowledge is not up to that of your colleagues." When she polled her African American classmates to see what their experiences were with this faculty member, she discovered that he also wrote similar comments on their write-ups.

Peer Support Remedies

The first step in coping with racism is to use the support system you already have in place. Talk with your friends and family so that you won't feel as isolated. Do not respond in anger to the perpetrator. Remember that you can't fight every battle and that your primary goal is to graduate and become a physician (success is the best revenge!).

Many of the students we talked to chose to use informal supports because they were worried about a "domino effect" if they reported faculty members. Recognizing that the incident is a function of the perpetrator's problems, not yours, goes a long way in helping you cope with racist incidents. Similarly, your peers may help you remember that the entire institution does not sympathize with the faculty or staff member's racial bias. These methods will help you through "minor" incidents.

If you choose to form a group to combat racism on campus, there should be two primary goals: (a) ensuring support of the victim and (b) scrupulous documentation of discrimination (Berrill, 1992). The welfare of the actual victim of the incident should be the foremost focus of your group. This support includes helping with, and abiding by, the victim's decision whether or not to publicize the incident. Emotional support, including reminding the student of the availability of counseling, is important because of the sense of isolation he or she may feel after a bias incident.

For its advocacy function, your group must set *clear goals* and establish strategic plans to ensure a unity of purpose among its members. You may find it useful to develop alliances with other minority or women's groups with similar concerns. Perpetrators may not discern between the groups as targets of future attacks. Advocacy groups should have a clear understanding of the institution's procedures for setting policy on race bias concerns. You must present the *documentation* you have gathered to the school's administration to assist in the development of these policies. If possible, victims willing to describe their experiences should make presentations to the administration officials. If the administration is not responsive, it may be necessary to seek legal action, involve the media, or demonstrate (Berrill, 1992).

One ongoing advocacy task of your group should be to *maintain a database* of known harassment and discrimination incidents. This can help establish that events are not isolated. It also will help your school's administration to set an agenda of increased awareness of the problems faced by minority group members on campus. Increased awareness alone may help prevent future race motivated incidents.

You may need to make several *recommendations* to the school administration—for example, increased minority faculty representation, enhancement of school security, support for affirmative action, and increased minority student involvement in administrative affairs (U.S. Commission on Civil Rights, 1990). You can also suggest an increase in resources to assess the need for formalized multicultural and mediation training on the campus.

The medical school administration will have to establish a balance between the constitutional protection of free speech and protection from racial harassment. There should be zero tolerance for any form of discrimination. They should encourage the reporting of bias incidents and develop clear policies and procedures for addressing them. The institution may need to develop task forces to collect data about incidents, develop a methodology for reporting the incidents, assist victims, discipline perpetrators, and educate the campus and the community at large (Berrill, 1992).

Legal Remedies

The federal government states that "racial discrimination is present when people are treated differently than others who are similarly situated because they are members of a specific race. It can occur when individuals are treated differently because of unalterable characteristics, such as physical features, indigenous to their race" (National Institute of Environmental Health Sciences, 1998). Explicit acts against you, such as racial slurs or violence, are not necessary to show discrimination. It may be sufficient to provide evidence of a pattern of questionable behavior.

What is your university's or hospital's official policy regarding racial discrimination? Are there reporting guidelines and remedies? Do the hospital's discrimination policies apply to medical students? What options are available to you as a student? These are questions you should consider before an incident occurs.

Many institutions have affirmative action (AA) or equal employment opportunity (EEO) complaint policies for employees. Similar policies are probably available from the Office of Student Affairs. On some campuses, a consultation session can be held with your faculty adviser. However, you must consider that the faculty adviser may be bound by policy to report any colleague that is suspected of such abuses to the AA/EEO office. In that instance, you might need to withhold the identity of the person if you do not want to start the formal complaint process. Because of issues of confidentiality and the protection of the rights of the accused, we suggest that you first exhaust the services available within the university system when seeking advice.

Complaints Recognized as Racial Discrimination at One Institution[2]

▶ 1. Consultation—A conference or meeting is held to give advice or to exchange views in order to resolve complaints without an investigation.

▶ 2. Informal complaint—A verbal complaint is initiated by an applicant, employee, or student with the AA/EEO office in which no written file is created.

▶ 3. Formal complaint—A written complaint is filed with the AA/EEO office leading to an investigation.

Unofficial advisory panels made up of faculty members, students, or staff may also exist in your medical school. Given their unofficial nature, these panels may not be bound by the same reporting restrictions your faculty adviser must follow. Unlike groups organized specifically for emotional support, this panel helps students sort information to assist their decision on how to proceed.

At some point, you may decide that working within the university system is ineffective or ill-advised. You may have no other choice but to seek a legal remedy to your situation.

Making Your Case

Several federal civil statutes apply and can result in compensatory and punitive damages in cases of racial discrimination and harassment. The commonly cited federal statutes and sections are based on the Civil Rights Act of 1964 and are outlined in Table 12.1. One key feature of the legislation is that damages can be awarded despite the existence of clearly stated university policies against discrimination.

When an antidiscrimination policy is in place in a hospital or university, it is designed to shield the institution from liability for the actions of a rogue employee. If the institution is successful in being dropped from the claim and leaves the individual perpetrator to stand alone in the action, damage recovery becomes difficult. Usually, an individual does not have the ability to pay significant monetary damages compared with the vast resources of an institution. You may need to review your state's vicarious liability statutes and common-law precedents with your attorney to determine the extent of the institution's culpability.

Table 12.2 reviews the federal criminal statutes that apply to racial discrimination. These laws essentially criminalize racially motivated acts of one person against another. These statutes are applicable only in certain circumstances because of a restricted list of activities over which the federal government can claim jurisdiction and prosecute. Given the limited applicability of many of the federal civil and criminal laws and potential difficulties of successfully naming an institution in a lawsuit, you must be able to present clear, objective evidence to support a discrimination claim.

What Are the Facts?

It is important that you gather evidence to corroborate the details of the incident(s) in question. Documentation includes careful recording of each

Table 12.1 Federal Civil Codes Against Racial Discrimination

Federal Statute	Statement of Law	Implications
Title VI of the 1964 Civil Rights Act (42 U.S.C. § 2000d)	No person in the United States shall, on the grounds of race . . . be excluded from participation in, be denied the benefits of, or be subjected to discrimination under any program or activity receiving Federal financial assistance.	A student victim who can show either intentional discrimination or disparate impact under Title VI can sue simply for experiencing racism; there does not need to be a specific violation of a university or hospital policy.
42 U.S.C. § 1981	All persons within the jurisdiction of the United States shall have the same right . . . to make and enforce contracts . . . to the full and equal benefit of all laws . . . and property as is enjoyed by white citizens.	If a Black victim is denied the same "property"-type advantages of a White person, the victim has a cause of action. Property in the legal sense can be a tangible or intangible thing capable of being owned or transferred.
42 U.S.C. § 1983	Every person who, under color of any statute, ordinance, regulation, custom, or usage, of any State of Territory or the District of Columbia, subjects, or causes to be subjected, any citizen of the United States or other person within the jurisdiction thereof to the deprivation of any rights, privilege, or immunities secured by the Constitution and laws, shall be liable to the party injured.	There does not need to be a stated policy against racism, just the violation of a guaranteed right. The limitation of the statute is that the wrongful action must be taken "under color" of state law. In other words, there has to be the appearance that the violation was acceptable under state law before recovery of damages under the Federal statute.
Title VII (42 U.S.C. § 2000e-2)	It is unlawful for an employer to discriminate on the basis of such individual's race, color, religion, sex or national origin. . . . It is illegal for two or more persons in any State or Territory to conspire . . . for the purpose of depriving, either directly or indirectly, any person or class of persons of the equal protection of the laws, or of equal privileges and immunities under the laws . . . in any case or conspiracy set forth in this section . . . whereby another is injured in his person or property, or deprived of having and exercising any right or privilege of a citizen of the United States, the party so injured or deprived may have an action for the recovery of damages.	Title VII applies to employers with 15 or more employees. Here, the courts recognize two types of racial discrimination: intentional and disparate treatment or impact. Again, an official organization antidiscrimination policy does not have to be in existence for the victim to recover damages.

Table 12.2   Federal Criminal Laws Against Racial Discrimination

Federal Law	Statement of Law	Implications
18 U.S.C. § 241 and18 U.S.C. § 242	Section 241 criminalizes the prohibited conspiracies found in 42 U.S.C. § 1985. 242 criminalizes acts against someone "on account of such person being an alien, or by reason of his color, or race," that deprive the victim "of any rights, privileges, or immunities secured or protected by the Constitution of laws of the United States . . ."	Section 241 provides a long laundry list of federally protected activities, but the history of § 242 indicates a very narrow construction of when federal agents can step in and prosecute.

incident, including names or descriptions of perpetrators, keeping photocopies of written material and tapes of incriminating speech from lectures or messages on answering machines. Your witnesses can be classmates, nurses, social workers, housekeeping staff, or possibly, patients. Obtain affidavits from anyone who can corroborate your claim. The evidence that you gather will assist your attorney with building your case.

In the case of an erroneous evaluation, it would be helpful to obtain written evaluations from the individual or faculty members that may refute the evaluation in question. Try to gather evidence that includes a direct reference to race or physical features "unique" to a race. For the student described above who stated that all the African American students had similar negative evaluations from a faculty member, evaluations should also be obtained. It will be crucial to compare them with those of her nonminority student counterparts to support the "different treatment in similar situations" claim.

It is also important to document the damages that you have incurred as a result of the racist act. This can be a lower grade than what should have been given, loss of a scholarship, dismissal from school, or emotional injury of the variety described earlier. If you were subjected to physical violence requiring medical treatment, obtain medical records and photographs of physical injuries. If poor grades are the results of discrimination, then it is crucial that a claim or inquiry begin immediately after this is suspected. Poor academic standing at the time of a claim makes it difficult to show that your action against the university was motivated by a quest for justice as opposed to a ploy for readmission or retaliation against the school.

Summary

Racism exists when one believes that race is the primary determinant of human traits and capacities. It is difficult to present statistically significant data to support a claim of racism against a particular faculty member. However, your speaking up in the event of questionable behavior by your colleagues or teachers may be the first step toward improving your school's ennui toward racially sensitive issues. Medical educators' willingness to explore their feelings and beliefs regarding race in order to create learning environments conducive to the development of all their students will make them better educators.

As a medical student today, you have access to a broad range of advice regarding your rights as a student and a U.S. citizen. The psychological or physical injuries that you sustain as a result of racial discrimination are recognized in federal courts as worthy of remuneration. Even though we encourage you to make a sincere effort to work within your institution's mechanisms to rectify the wrongs of particular individuals in the school, you still need to be aware of your legal rights and responsibilities should you seek recovery for damages from the courts.

Discussion Vignettes

The following stories were provided by medical students from around the country. Do you think the situations represent racial prejudice? What other information do you need to make a determination? Finally, how would you feel in these situations? What would you do? How would you advise a classmate?

Vignette 1. I was raised in a primarily White neighborhood in the North where my ethnic background was considered irrelevant by my neighbors and friends. In college, my clique was multiethnic. However, I went to medical school in the South. I was one of very few minorities in my class. In the first days when we were getting to know each other, only the minority students initiated conversations with me. The White students identified me as a person of color first and an individual second.

Vignette 2. I was preparing to take the National Board Examination. My aunt, who was my surrogate mother while I was away in medical school, became ill and died. When I wanted to postpone taking the board exam, my class faculty supervisor's only comment was, "Deal with your family today, but you know that gives you one less day to study when you start studying again." A White student in my class, in a similar situation, was given the option of not taking the exam but chose to take it anyway. A letter was placed in his file indicating that a poor score should be excused because he'd had a death in his family.

Vignette 3. It was my first day of my pediatrics rotation. We would be located primarily in two hospitals—a downtown urban university hospital that serves an often-indigent population and a suburban hospital with a more middle-class population. The attending compared the two patient populations. "A mother at University hospital may not know her baby's Apgar scores, where all the mothers at Suburban Hospital will. Mothers at University Hospital may not know about things like the baby's birth weight or medications. Mothers at Suburban Hospital will. . . . It's important to tell the mothers the importance of reading to their children. A lot of University hospital moms don't even own books. You pretty much won't have that problem at Suburban hospital, though. . . ." Students are listening with rapt attention. The attending asks, "So who do you think sees more head lice, University Hospital, or Suburban Hospital?" The students in unison respond, "University Hospital." The attending smiles broadly and says, "No, believe it or not, it's Suburban Hospital. You see, Black children just don't get lice . . . believe it or not."

Vignette 4. The lecturer asked, "How many of you feel that if a woman only wants to see a female gynecologist that she should be able to?" Most of the 75 students in the auditorium raised their hands. He then asked, "What if a woman wanted only to see a White gynecologist and not a Black one?" Two people raised their hands. The lecturer asked, "Why is it OK for a woman to discriminate against a male gynecologist and not a Black one?"

Vignette 5. A woman was one of the first students in her medical school through a program designed to increase the number of Native American students in medical schools in her region. On her arrival, the dean informed her that she would receive no special favors. He then assured her that she would have a difficult time. Her White colleagues readily identified the dean's behavior as "redneck racism." At the time of her graduation, the dean walked up to her and said, "Well, you finally made it."

Vignette 6. In a residency selection committee, a Caucasian female attending stated, "If I had to choose between a White man and a Black woman, I'd pick the woman because they're hardworking, reliable, and intelligent. For her to make it this far, she is bound to have overcome a lot of obstacles. . ."

NOTES

1. We wish to acknowledge the contribution of attorney Charles T. Smith II to this chapter in providing explanations of the federal antidiscrimination statutes and how they relate to potential damage recovery by medical students. We also thank the medical students and physicians who shared their stories with us.

2. Affirmative Action/EEO Complaint Policy, University of Medicine and Dentistry of New Jersey (www.umdnj.edu/oppmweb/00-01-35-55_00.html).

REFERENCES

Association of American Medical Colleges. (1987). *AAMC statement on medical education of minority group students.* Washington, DC: Author.

Association of American Medical Colleges. (1997). Medical school applicants, enrollment, and graduates from underrepresented minority groups, Table B6. In AAMC, *AAMC data book: Statistical information related to medical education.* Washington, DC: Author.

Bard, M., & Sangrey, D. (1979). *The crime victim's book.* New York: Basic Books.

Barnes, A., & Ephross, P. S. (1994). The impact of hate violence on victims: Emotional and behavioral responses to attacks. *Social Work, 39,* 247-251.

Berrill, K. T. (1992). Organizing against hate on campus: Strategies for activists. In G. M. Herek & K. T. Berrill (Eds.), *Hate crimes: Confronting violence against lesbians and gay men.* Newbury Park, CA: Sage.

Bright, C. M., Duefield, C. A., & Stone, V. E. (1998). Perceived barriers and biases in the medical education experience by gender and race. *Journal of the National Medical Association, 90,* 681-688.

Chun, K., & Zalokar, N. (1992). *Civil rights issues facing Asian-Americans in the 1990s.* Washington, DC: U.S. Commission on Civil Rights.

Dovidio, J. F., & Gaertner, S. L. (1986). Prejudice, discrimination and racism: Historical trends and contemporary approaches. In J. F. Dovidio & S. L. Gaertner (Eds.), *Prejudice, discrimination, and racism* (pp. 1-34). Orlando, FL: Academic Press.

Ellis, F. J. (1997, March/April). Color blind rulings derail diversity in medicine. *Academic Physician & Scientist, 1,* 12.

Garnets, L., Herek, G. M., & Levy, B. (1990). Violence and victimization of lesbians and gay men. *Journal of Interpersonal Violence, 5,* 366-383.

McLaughlin, K. A., & Brilliant, K. J. (1997). *A national bias crime prevention curriculum for middle schools.* Newton, MA: Education Development Center.

McLaughlin, K. A., Brilliant, K., & Lang, C. (1995). *National bias crimes training for law enforcement and victim assistance professionals.* Newton, MA: Education Development Center.

National Institute of Environmental Health Sciences, National Institutes of Health. (1998). s.nih.gov/oeeo/race.htm

Nebraska Advisory Committee to the U.S. Commission on Civil Rights. (1990). *Bigotry and violence on Nebraska's college campuses* (Summary report). Washington, DC: U.S. Commission on Civil Rights.

Roberts, J. (1995). *Disproportionate harm: Hate crime in Canada (1995)* (Working paper). kor.org/hweb/orgs/canadian/canada/justice/disproportionate-harm/

Sales, E., Baum, M.,& Shore, B. (1984). Victim readjustment following assault. *Journal of Social Issues, 40*(1), 117-136.

U.S. Commission on Civil Rights. (1990). *Bigotry and violence on American college campuses.* Washington, DC: Author.

Winton, A. S., Singh, N. N., & McAleavy, K. (1998). Perpetrators of racial violence and hatred. In A. Bellack & M. Hersen (Eds.), *Comprehensive clinical psychology: Vol 9. Applications in diverse populations.* Oxford, UK: Elsevier Science.

Afterword

The gray of that cool October morning was a perfect complement to the sense of gloom I felt as I entered the rather stark, sparsely furnished room. Seated behind a wooden table were two elderly gentlemen, one of whom beckoned to me to be seated. I knew the numbers. Of 160 students admitted to the medical school, a very limited number would be non-White. Would I be one of the "chosen?" As I approached the wooden chair, I sensed that a moment of truth had arrived.

During that medical school admissions interview over 40 years ago, I was asked if I thought that I might go to the rural South to take care of "poor colored people" when I completed medical school. That the institution was located in the urban North says volumes about the perspectives of the interviewers. Those were the behaviors and attitudes of the times. There were no advocates, no mentors, no affirmative action, and no minority affairs offices or personnel. "Quotas" were magical numbers representing the *maximum* (not minimum) number of minorities that could be admitted. Racism was alive and well.

There are those who would now deny the present reality of racism. After all, aren't there many more minority physicians these days? But one need only note the disparity in health care accessibility for members of the defined underrepresented minority groups to realize that the attitudes that reflect racism, both individual and institutional, still very much influence the manner in which we, as a nation, do business. And that reality, more than any other single factor, underscores the necessity for *Taking My Place in Medicine: A Guide for Minority Medical Students.*

Although this volume has been written primarily for minority medical students, nonminority students, faculty members, and administrators have much to gain from reading it as well. It is time for all of us, and particularly physicians, to recognize that our learning must include more than a passing knowledge of the many cultures in a diverse society. And where do we go from here? Perhaps the next volume of this book should outline techniques that would specifically address diversity training and multicultural competence within medical education. As a start, the Association of American Medical Colleges has recently established a task force to structure a Liaison Committee of Medical Education Standard on Diversity. Changing the medical education system to emphasize the treatment of diverse patient populations would necessarily help to change the culture of the health care system. The time is right. The social and economic imperatives are present. The health and well-being of all patients are at stake.

—Leonard E. Lawrence, M.D.

Associate Dean for Student Affairs and
Professor of Psychiatry, Pediatrics and Family Practice,
University of Texas Medical School at San Antonio

Author Index

Academic Affairs Human Resources, 141, 174
Achenbach, K., 111
Adams-Gaston, J., 82
Airhihenbuwa, C. O., 114
Alvord, L. A., 163, 170
American Academy of Family Physicians, 63, 76
Anderson, J., 191
Anderson, L. P., 108
Appleton, N., 162
Arlow, J. A., 104
Association of American Medical Colleges, 85, 141, 142, 158, 173, 174, 188, 199, 202
Atkinson, D. R., 115

Badt, K. L., 157
Bailey, E. J., 152
Baldwin, D., 111
Bard, M., 202
Barnes, A., 202
Barringer, F., 190
Baucom, J., 35
Baum, M., 202
Bazhanoodah, A., 160
Becker, H., 28
Becker, M., 144
Belfer, B., 107
Berlin, J., 155

Bernard, J., 34
Berrill, K. T., 201, 204, 205
Bindman, A., 66, 67, 196
Biondel, R., 162
Bland, I. J., 145
Blassingame, J., 149, 150, 151
Bloom, S., 10
Bonnett, A. W., 145
Bright, C. M., 199
Brilliant, K., 200, 202
Brown, J.H.B., 141
Bullock, S. C., 141, 150, 151
Burke, J., 155

Campbell, J., 10
Carson, B., 142
Carson, C., 150
Carter, J. H., 111, 145
Castaneda, A., 189
Chamberlain, M., 165
Christakis, D., 5, 9
Christenson, S., 182
Chun, K., 201
Clark, D. C., 111
Cohen, D., 82, 84, 85
Cohen, D. L, 189
Committee on Education Group, 24, 28
Conard, S., 111
Cooper, M., 115

Costello, R., 111
Courney, S., 191
Cozzens, L., 141
Crisp, J. E , 184
Curtis, J., 5

Daugherty, S. R., 64, 111
Davis, G., 87
Davis, L. E., 114
de los Santos, A. G., 89
Dickens, W. T., 82
Dickstein, L. J., 113
Diop, C. A., 140
Division of Community and Minority
    Programs, 142
Douglas, F. L., 145
Dovidio, J. F., 200
Draine, J., 110
Drake, M., 66, 67, 196
Dube, R., 155
Du Bois, W. E. B., 145
Duefield, C. A., 199
Duke University Center Medical Center
    Library, 139
Dumas, R., 146-147
Durmont, R., 161
Durrett, D., 157, 166
Duthu, B., 165

Eckenfels, E. J., 111
"Education Passports," 189
Eisenberg, J., 155
Elizondo, V., 105
Elkhanialy, H., 150
Ellis, F. J., 199
Ephross, P. S., 202
Epps, C. H., 139, 141
Erickson, F., 161
Escarce, J., 155

Fawcett, J., 111
Feldman, B., 111
Felton, J.C.M., 106, 122, 145
Fenichel, C., 86
Feudtner, C., 5, 9
Fine, P., 25
Finley, L., 149

Fischer, P., 111
Fitzpatrick, J. P., 191
Flaherty, J. A., 108
Folkman, S., 108, 109
Fontenot, W. L., 140
Forney, M., 111
Forney, P., 111
Frank, R. R., 144
Fraser, G. C., 149
Fullilove, M. T., 140, 141
Furlong, M. J., 115

Gaertner, S. L., 200
Galanti, G., 26, 85
Galloway, C. E., 163
Garb, H. N., 114
Garcia-Preto, N., 105
Garnets, L., 201
Garrod, A., 165
Garrow, D. J., 150
Geer, B., 28
Gersh, B., 155
Gill, G., 150
Ginsberg, M. B., 191
Gowda, K. K, 145
Grady, C., 82, 127, 129
Grebb, J. A., 87
Gregory, K., 151
Griffith, E., 106
Grumach, K., 66, 67, 195

Hale, J. E., 150
Hall, J., 9
Halpern, J., 104
Harding, V., 150
Harless, W., 155
Harry, B., 186
Havighurst, R. J., 161
Hawkins, M., 82, 84
Health Resources and Services
    Administration, 188
Helgeson, S., 9
Herek, G. M., 201
Hernstein, R. J., 82
Hine, D. C., 150
Hinz, L. D., 113
Hoffman, N. G., 111
Hoppe, S., 111

Hopwood v. Texas, 142, 174
Houston, E., 141, 150, 151
Hughes, E. C., 28
Hughes, P., 111

"Imhotep" Encyclopedia Britannica Online, 140
Iverson, Peter, 157

Jaynes, J. H., 35, 36
John, V., 163
Johnson, D. G., 139, 141

Kane, T. J., 82
Kaplan, H. I., 25, 26, 87
Kassebaum, D. G., 64
Kaugman, P., 189, 191
Keane, D., 66, 67, 196
Kerner, J., 155
Klein, S., 189, 191
Kleinfeld, J. S., 163
Kluckhohn, C., 161
Koepsell, T., 67
Komaromy, M., 66, 67, 195
Kyriazi, M., 111

Lago, C., 115
Lang, C., 202
Larimore, C., 165
Laung, E. K., 189
LaVeist, T., 84
Lazarus, R. S., 108, 109
Leake, B., 151
Lee, B., 35
Lesser, J., 115
Levy, B., 201
Lewis, D. C., 111
Linn, B. S., 108
Lombardi, V. Jr., 35
Lurie, N., 66, 67, 196
Lyans, N., 170
Lyans, O., 170
Lyons, A., 5

Maddux, J., 111
Magnuson, E., 111
Malidoma, P. S., 147
Massey, W. E., 148
Mbiti, J. S., 105, 140, 148

McAleavy, K., 200
McAuliffe, W. E., 111
McCreary, M. L., 145
McLaughlin, K. A., 200, 202
McMillen, M., 189, 191
Mechanic, D., 16
Meléndez, E., 189
Mercado, P., 115
Mikkanen, A. Q., 166
Mitchell, K., 85
Mohatt, G., 161
Morales, J., 189
Morantz, R., 86
Motley, C., 141
Murphey, C., 142
Murray, C., 82
Myers, A., 145
Myers, M. F., 31, 114

Nager, N., 145
National Institute of Environmental Health Sciences, 205
National Medical Association, 141
Nebraska Advisory Committee, 202
Ness, V., 161
Nieman, L., 96
Nivins, B., 107, 149, 150
Novack, D, 82, 85
Núñez, A., 28, 29, 30, 31, 32, 35, 36, 37, 84, 88, 89, 90, 98, 101

Ogbu, J. U., 191
Oren Lyons, O., 105

Pernell-Arnold, A, 149
Petrucelli, J., 5
Phileon, W. E., 163
Pinderhughes, E. B., 150
Pomerleau, C., 86
Post, D., 145
Poston, W. C., 115
Prewitt-Diaz, J. O., 186
Prieto, D. O., 82, 88
Proctor, E. K., 114
Pyskoty, C. E., 108

Raboteau, A., 105, 148
Ramirez, M., 189
Ramirez, R. R., 191

Ranier, K. L., 145
Reed, J., 189, 191
Reichard, G., 163
Reitzes, D., 150
Richards, J., 111
Richardson, D. A., 144
Richardson, R. C., 89
Richman, J. A., 108
Rico, M., 145, 147
Rippe, J., 107
Roberts, J., 202
Robinson, C. J., 149
Rohman, M., 111

Saadatmand, F., 145
Sadock, B.J., 25, 26, 87
Saha, S., 67
Sales, E., 202
Sangrey, D., 202
Santangelo, S., 111
Schuchert, M. K., 64
Schulman, K., 155
Schultze, C. L., 82
Schwartz, R., 111
Sedlacek, W. E., 82, 84, 88
Shea, S., 140, 141
Sheehan, D. V., 111
Shervington, D. O., 145
Shields, P., 23, 82, 149
Shore, B., 202
Simmons, H., 89
Simmons, M., 161
Singh, N. N., 200
Sistrunk, S., 155
Slavin, L.A.R., 145
Smith, D. G., 190
Smith, D. L., 106
Sobol, A., 117
Sokol, R. J., 144
Solomon, P., 110
Spurlock, J., 87
Stagnaro-Green, A., 145, 147
Stein, H. F., 28, 29, 98
Stephenson, J. J., 113
Sternberg, R. J., 82
Stone, V. E., 199

Strauss, A. C., 28
Strayhorn, G., 145
Sue, D., 115
Sue, D. W., 115
Szenas, P. L., 64

Taleghani, C., 155
Tatum, B. D., 122
Taylor, A. D., 63
Thompson, J., 115
Tracey, T. J., 88

U.S. Bureau of Labor Statistics, 188
U.S. Bureau of the Census, 188, 189
U.S. Commission on Civil Rights, 201, 204

Vaughan, A. L., 139, 141
Vranizan, K., 66, 67, 196

Watson, G., 87
Waugh, F., 84
Wax, D., 162
Wax, M., 162
Webb, C., 28, 30, 31, 32, 35, 36, 37, 82, 84,
    85, 88, 89, 90, 98, 101, 109, 149
Weddington, W., 145
Weissman, J., 111
Wells, K., 151
Whigham-Desir, M., 84
Williams, S., 155
Winton, A. S., 200
Wlodkowski, R. J., 35, 36, 191
Wright, C. A., 127, 128
Wright, S. D., 127, 128

Young, J. L., 106

Zalokar, N., 201
Zeldow, P., 64
Zeppa, R., 108

Subject Index

Academic competition, 13-14
Academic self-assessment, 88
Acceptance rates, of Native Americans, 173
Advisors, clinical, 56-57, 59
Affirmative action, 83, 141, 166, 174, 195, 199
African Americans, xvii, 151-152
　current status of, in medicine, 139-142
　history of, in medicine, 139-142
African Americans students, challenges to:
　Black physician identity, 145
　financial burdens, 147
　giving back to the community, 145-146
　racism, 144-145
　romantic relationships, 146-147
　socializing, 146
　See also Historically Black Medical
　　Schools (HBMSs)
African Americans students, success
　strategies for:
　awareness of history, 147-148
　controlling responses to racism, 149
　maintaining personal identity, 149-150
　organization, 151
　seeking help, 148
　spirituality, 148-149
Aggressiveness, 11
Alcohol abuse, 111-112
Always Being Right Answer Syndrome, 10
Always Being Right Syndrome, 10
American Association of Medical Colleges
　(AAMC), xvii, 141, 156, 157

American Medical Association (AMA), 141
Anatomy lab, 25
Ancillary personnel, 48
Assertiveness, 11
Attendance:
　classroom, 23-24
　lab, 25
Attending physician, 47
Attending rounds, 49

Bakke, Allen, 141
Balance:
　definition of, 29
　maintaining, 29-32, 61, 111
Bias crime, 200, 202
Bias incident, 200-201, 202-203
Blacks. *See* African Americans
Boricua/Latino Health Organization (BLHO),
　124, 194

Cadavers, 25-26
Carson, Ben, 142
Chain of command, 59
Charles R. Drew University of Medicine and
　Science, 142
Chart. *See* Medical record
Children, 133-134
Civil Rights Act of 1964, 206
Classroom attendance, 23-24

Clinical advisors, 56-57, 59
Clinical clerkships, 46-47
    daily routine during, 49-50
    defensive strategies during, 58-61
    potential problems during, 53-58
    student responsibilities during, 50-53
Clinical course evaluation, poor, 56-57, 60-61
Collaborative model, 9
Communication styles, 14-15
Community:
    choosing, 121-125
    definition of, 121
    finding religious, 125
Competition:
    definition of, 33
    managing, 33-34
Componential intelligence, 82
Computers, used in testing, 40
Confidentiality, 114-115
Confrontational learning, 10
Contextual intelligence, 82
Crumpler, Rebecca L., 140
Cultural racism, 200
Culture of medicine:
    hiding emotions in, 11-12, 104
    hierarchy of, 6, 9, 47-48, 75, 144-145
    language of, 16, 25
    racism in (*See* Racism)
    rules/structures of, 5-14, 7-8 (table)
    traditions of, 5-6
Curriculum vitae, 73

Dead bodies, cultural views toward, 26
Department of Minority Affairs, 125-127
Derham, James, 140
Desegregation, 141
Discrimination, 200
Doctoring styles, 9
Drake, Karen, 142
Dress, appropriate, 60, 73
Drew, Charles Richard, 151
Drug abuse, 111-112

Eastman, Charles, 157
Elders, Joycelyn, 142142
Emotional self-renewal, 103-105
Emotions, fear of, 11-12
Enrollment, medical schools:
    of Mexican Americans, 173-175
    of Puerto Ricans, 187

Ethnic identity, 4
Ethnic minority, xvii
Evaluation Commission of Foreign Medical
    Graduates (ECFMG), 173
Exclusionary tactics, 54-55
Exercise, 111
Experiential intelligence, 82

Faculty:
    at HBMSs, 144
    minority, 127, 129
    Puerto Rican, 187
Family:
    autonomy vs loyalty to, 130-131
    avoiding playing doctor to, 133
    balancing, 132-133, 182, 191-192
    children, 133-134
    overinvolvement with, 131-132
    parental overcommitment, 132
Fast study, 11
First-year resident. *See* Intern

H&P, written, 50-51
Harassment, 201
Hate crime, 200
Hate incident, 200-201
Health Resources and Services
    Administration (HRSA), xvii
Helle, Lorette, 157
High-control doctoring style, 9
High-maintenance support, 100
Hispanics, 173, 174
Historically Black Medical Schools
    (HBMSs), 142, 199
    academics at, 143-144
    socialization at, 143
Historically Black Schools, 83
Hopwood v. Texas, 142, 174
Howard University College of Medicine,
    142, 199

Imbalance, 29
Imhotep, 140
Imposter syndrome, 86-87
Income, 65
Individual racism, 200
Individual relaxation time, 31, 32
Institutional racism, 200
Intellectual self-renewal, 105

Intelligence, types of, 82
Intern, 47
Interpersonal relations, 12
Interviews. *See* Residency interviews
Intimacy, personal, 104-105
Irby, Edith Mae, 140
Isolation, 119-121, 159-160

Jemison, Mae C., 142
Journaling, 104

Kountz, Samuel Lee, 151

Lab attendance, 25
Lab partners, choosing, 24
Lee, Rebecca, 199
Letters of recommendation, 47, 72-73
Level playing field, 83
Life maintenance time, 31
Low-control doctoring style, 9

Mahone, Paula, 142
MCAT, 84-85
McKenzie, Taylor, 157
Medical record, 49, 51
Medical rules, understanding/interpreting,
    7-8 (table)
Medical training, historic lack of minority
    access to, 5
Meharry Medical College, 142, 199
Mental health support:
    ambivalence toward, 113-114
    choosing, 114-115
Mentors, 93, 127-128, 167
    definition of, 127
    evaluating relationship with, 129-130
    finding, 59-60, 128-129
    for Mexican American students, 183
Mestizos, 172
Mexican American students, challenges to:
    being perceived as foreigners,
        175-176
    losing ethnic identity, 176
    See also Microinsults
Mexican American students, success
    strategies for:
    commitment to succeeding, 181-182
    family support, 182
    government/private programs, 183

group support, 182
mentors, 183
Mexican Americans, xvii, 184
    history of, in medicine, 173-174
    racial diversity of, 173
Microinsults, 175-176
    dealing with, 182
    examples of, 177-181
    See also Racism
Minority, as a term, xviii
Minority affairs department, 125-127
Minority Affairs Office, 110
Minority faculty, 127, 129
Minority patients, serving, 66-69, 85-86,
    145-146, 167-168
Minority students, xiv
Mistakes, admitting to, 60
Morehouse College of Medicine, 142
Motivation:
    managing, 36-38
    reasons for lack of, 35-36
Myths about minorities:
    acting white, 85
    affirmative action dependency, 83
    as manipulative, 82-83
    lack of intelligence, 81-82
    minority patient care, 85-86
    poorly prepared, 83-84
    standardized tests problems, 84-85
Myths about minorities, impact of:
    imposter syndrome, 86
    survivor guilt, 87-88

NAACP. *See* National Association for the
    Advancement of Colored People
National Association for the Advancement of
    Colored People (NAACP), 141
National Board of Medical Examiners shelf
    exams, 39, 40
National Medical Association (NMA), 74,
    93, 141
National Minority Mentor Recruitment
    Network, 129
National Residency Matching Program,
    75-76
Native American students:
    giving back to the community and,
        167-168
    mentors/role models for, 167
    secrets of success for, 166-167

Native American students, challenges to:
    affirmative action backlash, 166
    communication styles, 163
    cultural taboos, 163-164
    dress/appearance differences, 159-160
    inadequate academic preparation,
        158-159
    isolation, 159
    learning differences, 162-163
    racism, 164-166
    social adjustment, 159-160
    tribal obligations, 164
    values differences, 161-162
Native Americans, xvii, 156
    current status of, in medical school, 158
    history of, in medicine, 156-157
    spirituality, 168
    tribal membership, 156, 157, 169
NBME shelf exams, 39, 40
Networking, 128
NMA. *See* National Medical Association
Nursing personnel, 48

Onesimus, 140
Oral presentations, 60
Orientation, student, 23
Outpatient activities, 50

Patients, 48
    minority, 66-69, 85-86, 145-146, 167-168
    personal relationships with, 54
    rejection of student by, 53-54
Peck, David J., 140
Peer support, 203-205
Personal identity, developing, 3-5
Personal needs, evaluating:
    concrete advice sources, 99
    emotional/social needs, 99
    life maintenance, 99
    spiritual, 99
    time, 98
Personal statement, 73
Physical self-renewal, 107
Physician, attending, 47
Physician identity:
    creating, 4-5
    creating Black, 145
Playing the game, 6, 13-14
Power and influence, of doctors, 9-10
Prematriculation programs, 22-23

Prophylaxis, 108-109
Proposition 209 (California), 141, 174
Pseudosupport, 100
Puerto Rican students, challenges to:
    acculturation, 189-190
    communication skills, 190
    educational debt, 193
    family commitments, 191-192
    high dropout rate, 191
    isolation, 191
    lack of educational system support,
        193-194
    negative educational experiences,
        190-191
    poverty, 189
Puerto Rican students, secrets of success,
    194-195
Puerto Ricans, xvii, 195
    Commonwealth, 187
    current status of, in medicine, 187-188
    history of, in medicine, 187
    Mainland, 187
Punctuality, 60

Quotas, 141

Race, concept of, 184n1
Racial discrimination:
    federal criminal codes against, 206, 207
        (table)
    federal criminal laws against, 206, 208
        (table)
    gathering evidence for cases of, 206, 208
Racism:
    cultural, 200
    definition of, 198
    historical background, 199-200
    individual, 200
    institutional, 200
    managing response to, 93-94
    on campus, 201-202
    phases of reaction to, 202-203
    psychology of, 200-201
    toward African Americans, 144-145
    toward Native American students,
        164-166
    See also Microinsults
Racism, intervention strategies:
    legal remedies, 205-206
    peer support, 203-205

Residency application process:
    dean's letter, 72
    deciding where to apply, 70
    letters of recommendation, 72-73
    personal statement, 70-72
Residency interviews:
    appropriate dress for, 74
    inappropriate questions during, 75
    minority interviewer, 75
    punctuality, 74
    travel for, 74
Role models, 145, 167
Roundmanship, 10
Rounds, attending, 49

Sample conflicts, 17-20
SAT, 84
Scheduling time, 31-32
Scientific objectivity, 11-12
"Scut," 51
Self-appraisal, 88-94
    as different from academic self-
        assessment, 88
    initial steps in, 89-90
    interpreting clinical input, 90-93
    managing response to criticism/racism,
        93-94
Self-assessment, academic, 88
Self-renewal, finding:
    emotional, 103-105
    intellectual, 105
    physical, 107
    social, 105
    spiritual, 105-106
Smith, James M., 140
Social self-renewal, 105
Socratic teaching method, 25, 55-56
Specialty, choosing, 63-69
Spiritual self-renewal, 105-106
Spirituality, 99, 125, 148-149, 168
Stamina, necessity for, 13
Stereotypes, 200
Stress, coping with:
    bringing in outside perspective, 110
    by planned, limited escape, 110-111
    effect change to, 110
    recognizing stress, 108, 109
    using intervention, 108, 109-110
Student National Medical Association
    (SNMA), 122, 124, 148, 194

Student orientation, 23
Student responsibilities:
    assigned patients, 50-51
    expectations about, 52-53
    self-directed learning, 52
    teamwork, 51
Study habits, 26-27
Sub cortical utilization of time (Scut), 51
Subintern, 48
Substance abuse, 111-112
Sullivan, Louis, 151
Support:
    by family, 182
    mental health, 113-115
    obstacles to getting, 101-103
    peer, 203-205
    types of, 100-101
Supreme Court, 141, 142
Surgical procedures, assisting with, 49
Survivor guilt, 87-88

Teaching conferences, 50
Teaching resident, 47
Time:
    prioritizing, 31-32
    structured, 49-50
    unstructured, 50
Time constraints, 12, 16
Tribal membership, 156, 157, 169

Underrepresented minority (URM),
    increasing, 141
University of Arkansas, 140, 141
U.S. Medical Licensure Examination
    (USMLE), 39
    computers and, 40
    failing grade, 43
    format of, 40
    hindrances to studying for, 41-42
    preparing your mind-set for, 40-43
    reviewing for, 39-40
    strategies for taking, 43

Verbal assault, 201
Verbal communication, types of, 14-15

Work rounds, 49

About the Editor

Carmen Webb, MD, is Adjunct Assistant Professor of Psychiatry at MCP Hahnemann School of Medicine (MCPHU) and is currently in private practice in Dallas, Texas. She received her BS at Yale University, her medical degree from Southwestern Medical School, and her residency training at Hahnemann University. Throughout her career, she has been devoted to promoting medical student well-being. From 1992 to 1999, she served as Assistant Professor of Psychiatry and established the first Medical Student Mental Health Service at MCPHU. As director, she ensured the provision of confidential individual, group, and psychopharmacological treatment. She also codeveloped a curriculum and teaches courses and workshops to help minority and other students develop tools needed to survive the medical school culture. She recently assisted in building a framework for the service's expansion to a comprehensive well-being program.

Dr. Webb is the Principal Investigator of a multi-institutional research study evaluating the psychosocial characteristics and skills predictive of improved academic performance in medical school across race and gender. The research has been supported by grants from the Healthcare Resources Foundation and the Christian R. Mary F. Lindback Foundation. She served for seven years on the Admissions Committee at MCPHU and has been a consultant to a U.S. Medical Licensing Exam Preparation Program and to the Minority Affairs Program, assisting them in determining predictors of performance and support needs for minority students. She has made multiple presentations and published articles regarding predictors of medical school performance beyond standardized tests.

Very active in her community, Dr. Webb chaired the Board of Exodus to Excellence for six years (since its inception). This program stimulates minority students' achievement in math and science. She is married to a fine physician and is the mother of two wonderful boys.

About the Contributors

Cheryl S. Al-Mateen, MD, is a Forensic Child and Adolescent Psychiatrist on the faculty at the Medical College of Virginia at Virginia Commonwealth University in Richmond. She is also a faculty associate at the Institute for Law, Psychiatry and Public Policy at the University of Virginia. She received her undergraduate and medical degrees from Howard University and completed her psychiatric training at Hahnemann University in Philadelphia. Her research interests include the effects of all forms of violence on children and adolescents. She has publications and presentations related to this area as well as in the areas of cultural competence, sexuality, and the identity development and mental health of African American women. She is married to her coauthor and is the mother of two great children.

Kevin Bakeer Al-Mateen, MD, MSHA, is a Neonatologist on the faculty at the Medical College of Virginia at Virginia Commonwealth University (MCV of VCU) in Richmond. He did his undergraduate work at the University of California at Davis and received his medical degree from Howard University College of Medicine. He completed his Pediatric residency at St. Christopher's Hospital for Children in Philadelphia and his Neonatology fellowship at MCV of VCU. He has also received a master's degree in health administration from VCU. His research and publications relate to the treatment of respiratory disease and illness in newborns. He is also interested in the history and development of physician managers. He has been a member of the Committee on the Status of Women and Minorities in Medicine at VCU as well as serving as faculty adviser to residents and medical students. He is married to his coauthor and is the father of two great children.

Lori Arviso Alvord, MD, is Associate Dean of Student Affairs and Minority Affairs at Dartmouth Medical School and an Assistant Professor of Surgery. She did her medical training and residency/chief residency in general surgery at Stanford Medical School. Prior to this position, she worked six years with the Public Health Service as a surgeon for the Navajo and Zuni tribes in Arizona and Gallup, New Mexico. She is an enrolled member of the Navajo Tribe and lived in Navajo communities growing up (through high school). She is the first woman surgeon of her tribe. One of the most accomplished Native Americans in medicine today, she has oversight responsibility for the Offices of Student Affairs, Admissions, Financial Aid, the Registrar, the Advising Dean's Program, and Minority Affairs.

Miguel A. Bedolla, MD, PhD, MPH, is Associate Professor of Family Practice at the University of Texas Health Science Center in San Antonio and is also the Charles Miller, MD, Professor of Medical Ethics at St. Mary's University. He is the Director of the South Texas/Border Region Partnership for Health Professions Education, the South Texas/Border Region Partnership of Magnet High Schools/Programs for the Health Professions, and the Health Career Opportunities Program. He is a consulting ethicist with the University Health System. He does research on the historical and philosophical foundations of medical ethical codes, which has been published in *Insight: A Journal of Lonergan Studies* and *Médico Interamericano.* He has a B.A. in history from St. Mary's University, an MD from the Universidad de Nuevo Leon, a PhD from Ohio State University, and an MPH from the University of Texas. He is especially committed to creating opportunities for minority applicants to attend the medical schools of Texas.

George C. Gardiner, MD, FAPA, has most recently served as Clinical Director of the Dr. Warren E. Smith Health Centers in Philadelphia, a community-based comprehensive health center. A graduate of Tufts University School of Medicine, he is board certified in internal medicine and in psychiatry and has been involved in recruiting and retaining medical students over the last 30 years. His experience has included recruiting medical students; teaching them internal medicine and psychiatry; offering them academic counseling, career counseling, and psychotherapy; and organizing and maintaining support services for them. From 1989 until 1998, he was Associate Dean for Minority Affairs in what is now the MCP Hahnemann School of Medicine. In addition, during that time, he held the position of Associate Provost for Minority Affairs of Allegheny University of the Health Sciences and was responsible for establishing a complex set of programs designed to recruit minority students into the health professions. Much of this work entailed the individual career counseling of minority students interested in the health professions.

Margarita Hauser Gardiner, MD, is currently employed by a major pharmaceutical firm as a drug safety monitor. She is an honor graduate of Howard University and of the Medical College of Pennsylvania and is board certified in Internal Medicine and Rheumatology. She is a member of the American College of Physicians and is a fellow of the American College of Rheumatology. She was Assistant Professor of Medicine at the Medical College of Pennsylvania, now MCP Hahnemann School of Medicine, for six years and is now a member of the volunteer faculty. Her teaching responsibilities have included introductory courses in clinical medicine, third- and fourth-year medicine clerkships, fourth-year rheumatology electives, bioethics, and problem-based learning. She has been a clinical preceptor for second-, third-, and fourth-year medical students and was an academic adviser for five years. She continues to mentor premedical and medical students.

Maria Soto-Greene, MD, is Acting Associate Dean for Special Programs at the New Jersey Medical School and principal investigator of a federally funded program whose ultimate goal is to increase the number of Hispanic/Latino physicians who in turn will affect the health of their communities. This program also addresses the need for increased representation of Hispanic faculty members in medical school as well as the development of culturally competent curricula. She is responsible for the implementation of this and other pipeline education programs designed to increase the number of minority and disadvantaged students entering all of the health professions, including medicine. Her work with pipeline programs at the New Jersey Medical School was recently published in a recent issue of *Academic Medicine.* Board certified in internal medicine, critical care, and emergency medicine, she has 16 years experience as a faculty member involved with minority issues. She feels uniquely qualified to address issues related to Puerto Rican medical students as a Puerto Rican herself and because of her experience in providing the academic and nonacademic support to these students for so many years.

Morris Hawkins, Jr., PhD, is Associate Professor of Cell Biology and Molecular Genetics and Special Assistant to the Dean of the College of Medicine at Howard University. He received a PhD in Genetics from Howard University, and his postgraduate training includes Somatic Cell/Human/Neurogenetics at Yale University School of Medicine, Neurobiology at the Marine Biological Laboratory, health professions education leadership development at the University of Illinois Health Science Center, health management education at the Association of American Medical Colleges, and human molecular genetics at the National Cancer Institute. He has published articles in the fields of Biochemical and Somatic Cell Genetics dealing with gene mapping and regulation as well as recent works investigating the treatment of breast cancer. He has also published several articles on issues related to medical student matriculation, and he continues to serve as research adviser to undergraduate, medical, and doctorate students. He is president of the Shiloh Church Family Life Center Foundation Board of Directors and Faculty Athletics Representative to the National Collegiate Athletic Association and Mid-Eastern Athletic Conference for Howard University. He is very active in community service and is a life member of Alpha Phi Alpha Fraternity, Inc. He is involved in physical fitness, photography, and the cultural arts.

Ann Hill, MEd, obtained her BA from West Virginia University and her MS in guidance and counseling from Ohio University. As past Director of Minority Affairs at MCP Hahnemann School of Medicine, she was an advocate for minority students, providing personal and educational support and counseling. As an Assistant Professor and Assistant Director of Admissions at Cheyney University of Pennsylvania, she directed the Freshman Studies Program, in which she assisted students in developing strategies for academic success. She also directed the program for high-risk undergraduate students, and taught a seminar in "How to Be Successful in College."

Juan C. Martínez, EdD, is Senior Educational Planner at UMDNJ—New Jersey Medical School where he conducts individual and group cognitive development sessions, particularly with first- and second-year students, and coordinates support services such as individual tutorial services and the Biochemistry Group Tutorial Program. He also contributes to the planning and implementation of the Medical Educators in Training (METs) program in physiology and the Freshman Introduction to Resources, Skills and Training (FIRST) summer program. A graduate of Boston University, Graduate School of Education, he has over 20 years of experience in student academic advisement and development. Before bringing his expertise to medical education, he served as Program Specialist for the New Jersey Department of Higher Education. His community involvement includes presentations at local colleges and community educational centers to promote health and science professions and academic excellence. He is the secretary of the statewide Hispanic Association for Higher Education of New Jersey (HAHENJ, Inc.) and is an English as a second language (ESL) volunteer teacher in his community.

Ana E. Núñez, MD, is Assistant Professor of Medicine, Assistant Dean for Generalism, Director of the Women's Health Education Program, and Medical Director for the Physician Assistant Program at MCP Hahnemann School of Medicine. She received her medical degree and residency training at Hahnemann University in Philadelphia, Pennsylvania. Her postgraduate training includes a medical education fellowship in the Primary Care Faculty Development Program at Michigan State University in 1993 and a Health Services Research fellowship at the Association of American Medical Colleges in 1995. She is currently the principal investigator in a U.S. Department of Education Fund for Improvement of Post-Secondary Education Disseminating Proven Reforms Grant in Women's Health Education and a grant for health provider cultural competency for women of color who have HIV disease within the Institute of Women's Health Center for Excellence. She also serves as the editor of comprehensive women's health case studies series titled, *Healthy Women, Healthy Lives: Women's Health Across the Lifespan.* As a nationally recognized expert on cultural diversity and cross-cultural communication, she has presented at numerous conferences and served on national advisory's addressing cultural diversity training and its impact on health care. She is currently an invited member to the National Advisory to the Robert Wood Johnson Minority Medical Education Program.

Stephanie Smith is currently attending her third year at Virginia Commonwealth University's Medical College of Virginia. She completed her first two years of medical education at MCP Hahnemann School of Medicine, where she received recognition as a Humanities Scholar. At that institution, she participated in activities such as the SNMA, Holistic Medicine Society, Pen Friends, and several outreach programs. She is also the principal investigator of a project examining the academic and personal guidance that practicing physicians of color might offer to minority medical students to help them succeed in medical school.

BAKER & TAYLOR